Diagnosis and
Management
Muscle Disease

Neurologic Illness:
DIAGNOSIS & TREAMENT

EDITOR-IN-CHIEF
Michael I. Weintraub, M.D.
New York Medical College
Valhalla, NY

Hysterical Conversion Reactions
Michael I. Weintraub

Infectious Diseases of the Central Nervous System
Richard A. Thompson and John R. Green, eds.

Diagnosis and Management of Muscle Disease

Albert P. Galdi, M.D.

Georgetown University Hospital
Washington, D.C.

Director EMG Laboratory
National Naval Medical Center
Bethesda, Maryland

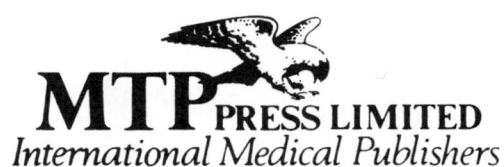

MTP PRESS LIMITED
International Medical Publishers

Published in the UK and Europe by
MTP Press Limited
Falcon House
Lancaster, England

Published in the US by
SPECTRUM PUBLICATIONS, INC.
175-20 Wexford Terrace
Jamaica, NY 11432

ISBN-13: 978-94-011-6337-8   e-ISBN-13: 978-94-011-6335-4
DOI: 10.1007/978-94-011-6335-4

Dedication

This book is affectionately dedicated to my parents, my wife, Anna, and my children, Albert and Marisa.

Preface

Neurologists and non-neurologists alike can no longer ignore diseases of the neuromuscular system. The old dogma that these disorders are both uncommon and untreatable has lost its validity. Recent technological advances have enabled us to study more precisely muscle and nerve anatomy, physiology and biochemistry. Because of this progress, we are now recognizing new neuromuscular diseases as well as diagnosing more subtle cases of myasthenia gravis, myotonia, and metabolic myopathies. Treatment of the neuromuscular diseases has also undergone dramatic change based on new discoveries in the fields of immunology and pharmacology. No longer are myotonia, periodic paralysis, and malignant hyperthermia untreatable medical curiosities. No longer are cases of steroid-unresponsive myositis given up as hopeless. Because of all these advances, non-surgical physicians and especially neurologists must update their knowledge regarding the neuromuscular disorders.

This book, it is hoped, will help such clinicians in dealing with this task. Emphasis has been placed on the diagnosis and management of these disorders rather than on their pathophysiology. The more uncommon diseases and those of uncertain existence have been omitted purposely and left to the larger and more encyclopedic reference works.

Chapter 1 discusses the clinical symptoms and signs of muscle disease and is designed to enable the reader to formulate a differential diagnosis on the basis of the patient's history and physical examination. Chapter 2 describes the important laboratory tests which will further aid the clinician in diagnosing the patient with neuromuscular problems. Chapters 3 through 11 serve as reference material and elaborate on specific muscle and neuromuscular junction disorders.

Contents

Chapter 8

Inflammatory Myopathies   **135**

Chapter 9

Disorders of Muscle Energy Metabolism and Mitochondria   **159**

Chapter 10

Neuromuscular Manifestations of Endocrine Dysfunction   **191**

Chapter 11

Toxic Myopathies   **205**

Index   **235**

ACKNOWLEDGMENTS

Much of the material contained reflects the teachings and philosophy of Dr. W. King Engel to whom I am greatly indebted. I am also grateful to the members of the Departments of Neurology at Georgetown University Hospital (Washington, D.C.) and National Naval Medical Center (Bethesda, Maryland). A final note of appreciation is expressed to Dr. Vernon Armbrustmacher of the Armed Forces Institutes of Pathology who graciously provided some of the histologic material contained within the text.

Diagnosis and Management Muscle Disease

CHAPTER 1

Clinical Assessment of the Patient with Neuromuscular Complaints

SYMPTOMS AND SIGNS OF NEUROMUSCULAR DISEASE

SYMPTOMS OF NEUROMUSCULAR DISEASE

History Taking/Family History

Proper evaluation of the patient with neuromuscular complaints begins with a carefully obtained family history as well as with a detailed account of the present illness. For the busy physician, listening to a patient's story often filled with inappropriate details, can be a frustrating and time-comsuming venture. However, it is the history, and to a lesser extent, the physical findings that determine the direction of the diagnostic evaluation. Therefore the time spent in talking with the patient is often a well-rewarded investment.

A detailed family history may be particularly important when dealing with a suspected neuromuscular disorder. The patient's statement that there is no family history of muscle disease cannot be casually accepted. Many neuromuscular syndromes produce such mild manifestations that the affected family members are unaware of their deficits. This is especially true in families with myotonic atrophy and the morphologically distinct myopathies. The importance of the family history when dealing with neuromuscular diseases is further emphasized in a recent report from the Mayo Clinic (Dyck et al, 1981). Over forty percent of patients referred there for further evaluation of undiagnosed peripheral nerve disease were subsequently found to have hereditary neuropathies. This diagnosis was made possible only after detailed questioning and examination of family members. Therefore, whenever possible, it is advantageous to examine all family members or at least see pictures of them.

Family history may also be important when the physician is confronted with unusual symptoms. For example, the patient who describes episodic bouts of total paralysis is often casually dismissed as a malingerer or a hysteric. However, if the family history uncovers relatives with similar problems, the diagnosis of a periodic paralysis becomes a strong consideration.

Because the number and diversity of diseases of muscles greatly exceed the number of symptoms and signs by which they express themselves clinically, different diseases share certain common symptoms. By far the most frequently encountered symptoms are weaknesses and muscle discomfort. These will be discussed below.

Weakness

Probably the most commonly presented complaint of patients with neuromuscular dysfunction is weakness. It is important to analyze such a complaint as to its anatomic distribution (proximal versus distal, with or without involvement of selective cranial nerve musculature), and to the time course. All muscles are not equally susceptible to disease despite the apparent similarity of their structure. In fact, practically no disease affects all muscles of the body and each disease has as one of its features a characteristic topography within the musculature. It should be possible after obtaining the history to predict which muscle groups are involved in the disease process. The patient with neuromuscular disease may describe the insidious development of difficulty climbing stairs, arising from a chair or a squatting position, or in raising the arms above the horizontal plane. These complaints reflect hip and shoulder girdle weakness. Many neuromuscular disorders, including polymyositis, endocrine myopathies, limb-girdle dystrophy, sarcoid myopathy, acid maltase deficiency, Eaton-Lambert syndrome, carnitine deficiency, and myopathies induced by steroids and ethanol abuse, begin with selective proximal weakness. Hip and shoulder girdle weakness are also found in myasthenia gravis, "ragged-red" fiber disease, and facioscapulohumeral and oculopharyngeal dystrophies, but in these illnesses prominent cranial musculature dysfunction (ptosis, diplopia and/or dysphagia) customarily precedes or accompanies the proximal limb weakness. Keep in mind, however, that not all proximal weakness reflects muscle or neuromuscular junction disease. Primary neurogenic disorders including the spinal muscular atrophies and proximal neuropathies may also produce predominant girdle weakness (see Table 1-1). Suspect these entities when there is a history of concomitant sensory abnormalities, autonomic dysfunction, early muscle wasting, and/or muscle twitches (fasciculations).

Loss of strength in the muscles of the distal upper extremities results in difficulty turning doorknobs and jar lids, and buttoning shirts. Stumbling over small objects and twisting of the ankles when walking on uneven surfaces suggest distal lower extremity weakness. Such problems more often indicate neuro-

Table 1-1. Neurogenic Causes of Proximal Weakness

Anterior Horn Cell Disease	Proximal Neuropathies
spinal muscular atrophy polio	Guillain-Barré syndrome porphyric neuropathy diabetic amyotrophy some toxic neuropathies paraneoplastic neuropathies plexopathies

genic (i.e., peripheral neuropathies and anterior horn cell disease) rather than myopathic disease.   However, several muscle disorders, including myotonic atrophy, inclusion body myositis, adult-onset rod disease, distal muscular dystrophy, and type I fiber hypotrophy, are also characterized by selective distal involvement (see Table 4-1). A history of other symptoms of peripheral nerve disease (sensory abnormalities, dysautonomia, fasciculations, etc.) is helpful in excluding these disorders.

Dysfunction of cranial nerve musculature produces a number of characteristic symptoms (see Table 1-2) and such involvement may provide important clues as to the etiology of the neuromuscular syndrome. In some diseases there is prominent and widespread dysfunction of cranial musculature. This is best exemplified by myasthenia gravis, botulism, and mitochondrial myopathies (i.e.,

Table 1-2. Characteristic Symptoms of Weakness in Specific Muscle Groups

Symptom	Site of Muscle Weakness
droopy lids (nicknamed "sleepy")	levators of eyelids
blurred or double vision	extraocular muscles
inability to whistle, drink through a straw, or blow up a balloon	facial muscles
hoarseness	laryngeal muscles
slurred speech	palatal, lingual, labial or pharyngeal muscles

uncontrolled snapping back of head
    when car decelerated or difficulty
    lifting head off pillow
	neck flexors

problems holding hair dryer over head or putting hair in rollers	shoulder girdle
difficulty turning door knobs and jar lids	distal upper extremities
difficulty getting out of a chair, climbing stairs, or rising from squat	hip girdle
waddling gait	hip abductors
problems going down stairs	knee extensors
tripping up stairs or on uneven ground	ankle dorsiflexors

Table 1-3. Topography of Cranial "Nerve" Involvement in Neuromuscular Diseases

Symptom/Sign	Muscle	NMJ	Neurogenic
ocular palsies/ ptosis	mitochondrial myopathies trichinosis some morphologically distinct myopathies hyperthyroid myopathy (usually no ptosis) myotonic atrophy (ptosis only) oculopharyngeal dystrophy (ptosis only)	myasthenia gravis botulism	Guillain-Barré (Fisher variant) diphtheric neuropathy cranial nerve arteritis brainstem/parasellar tumors chronic meningitis drugs/toxins Möbius syndrome
facial diplegia	facioscapulohumeral dystrophy myotonic atrophy some morphologically distinct myopathies mitochondrial myopathies	myasthenia gravis botulism	Guillain-Barré sarcoidosis Möbius syndrome motor neuron disease tumors Melkerson-Rosenthal syndrome cranial nerve arteritis
dysarthia dysphagia	myotonic atrophy myositis oculopharyngeal dystrophy mitochondrial myopathies	myasthinia gravis botulism	Guillain-Barré diphtheric neuropathy motor neuron disease syrinx cranial nerve arteritis tumors at base of brain chronic meningitis

Table 1-4. No Cranial "Nerve" Involvement

Muscle	NMJ	Neurogenic
Duchenne/Becker X-linked dystrophies adult-onset rod disease adult-onset acid maltase deficiency periodic paralysis steroid myopathy (atrophy) alcohol myopathy central core disease distal myopathy (dystrophy)	Eaton-Lambert syndrome	spinal muscular atrophies acquired/familial peripheral neuropathies

"ragged-red" fiber disease). In these disorders, ptosis, ophthalmoplegia, facial diplegia, dysarthria, and dysphagia are characteristically early and prominent manifestations. In other diseases there is more selective impairment of cranial musculature so that in oculopharyngeal dystrophy, for example, there is ptosis and dysphagia without ophthalmoparesis and facial weakness. In myositis the pattern is one of sparing extraocular and facial muscles with severe involvement of pharyngeal muscles. In still other myopathies there is no cranial involvement (i.e., periodic paralysis, Eaton-Lambert syndrome, Duchenne's muscular dystrophy) despite severe affliction of limb and girdle musculature (see Tables 1-3 and 1-4).

The time course is also an important characteristic when sorting out the causes of neuromuscular weakness. Weakness evolving rapidly over hours or days may be the presenting manifestation of a number of primary muscle or junction disorders. The periodic paralysis, myasthenia gravis, botulism, tick paralysis, systemic carnitine deficiency, and acute alcohol myopathy may produce the picture of rapidly evolving symmetric weakness without sensory abnormalities. Diseases of the anterior horn cells (i.e., polio), of peripheral nerves (i.e., Guillain-Barré syndrome), and of spinal cord (i.e., compressive myelopathy) are also capable of producing acutely symmetric weakness. These syndromes, however, can usually be distinguished and differentiated on the basis of accompanying clinical manifestations and laboratory studies. Fasciculations and spinal fluid pleocytosis help to incriminate polio as the culprit in such cases. Early areflexia, autonomic dysfunction, and sensory abnormalities localize the problem to the peripheral nerves, while incontinence, hyperreflexia, Babinski signs, and a sensory level implicate a extramedullary cord lesion (see Figure 1-1).

Other features in the time course of weakness may occasionally provide helpful clues. A patient who is strong on awakening in the morning, but loses strength in the later hours of the day, is a likely victim of myasthenia gravis. On the other hand, if the "weakness' is greatest on arising and improves after a

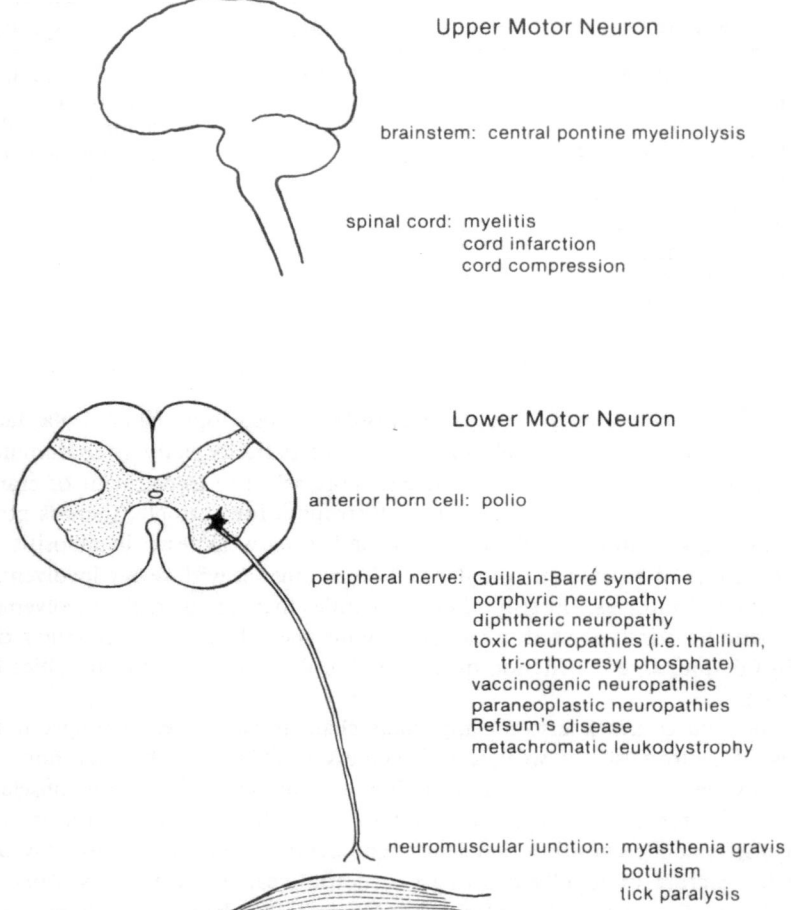

Upper Motor Neuron

brainstem: central pontine myelinolysis

spinal cord: myelitis
cord infarction
cord compression

Lower Motor Neuron

anterior horn cell: polio

peripheral nerve: Guillain-Barré syndrome
porphyric neuropathy
diphtheric neuropathy
toxic neuropathies (i.e. thallium,
tri-orthocresyl phosphate)
vaccinogenic neuropathies
paraneoplastic neuropathies
Refsum's disease
metachromatic leukodystrophy

neuromuscular junction: myasthenia gravis
botulism
tick paralysis

muscle: periodic paralysis
myositis
systemic carnitine deficiency

Figure 1-1.   Differential diagnosis of rapidly evolving symmetric weakness.

warm-up period, the Eaton-Lambert syndrome or a myotonic disorder should be suspected.

A rare patient may complain of exercise-induced weakness associated with the passage of dark tea-colored urine (myoglobinuria). With such a constellation of symptoms a problem of muscle energy metabolism (i.e., McArdle's disease) must be considered. Of course there are many other causes of myoglobinuria

Table 1-5. Causes of Myoglobinuria

excessive muscle activity
   voluntary, i.e., long distance running
   involuntary, i.e., status epilepticus, tetanus, electroshock therapy
isechemic or crush injuries to muscle
drugs (clofibrate, barbiturates, heroin) and toxins (alcohol, snake venom)
salt and water imbalances (hypokalemia, hypernatremia, acidosis)
infections and fevers
disorders of muscle energy metabolism
   disorders of glycogen/glucose metabolism (myophosphorylase deficiency,
      phosphoglycerate kinase deficiency, phosphoglycerate mutase deficiency,
      lactic acid dehydrogenase deficiency).
   disorders of lipid metabolism (carnitine palmityl transferase deficiency)
   others: malignant hyperthermia/neuroleptic malignant syndrome
other myopathies
   myositis
idiopathic

(See Table 1-5), the most common of which are excessive muscle activity, muscle trauma, and acute alcohol myositis (Grabow et al, 1982).

Muscle Discomfort

Muscle discomfort (cramps, twitching, soreness, and stiffness) commonly accompanies neuromuscular disturbances (see Table 1-6). Contrary to popular belief, the majority of people with cramps do not have primary muscle disease. Most cramps are of a benign nature (i.e., related to exertion and/or mild salt depletion). However, patients with peripheral neuropathies (especially familial neuropathies), anterior horn cell diseases, hypothyroid myopathy, and disorders of muscle energy metabolism may also experience severe muscle cramps. In the disorders of muscle glucose metabolism, the cramps are electrically silent in contrast to the usual high voltage rapid discharges of ordinary cramps observed by electromyography. For this reason they are more correctly referred to as (true) contractures. (Fixations of limb posture due to fibrosis of muscle and periarticular tissues are pseudocontractures.)

Painful, tender muscles may be a prominent symptom of inflammatory or toxin induced myopathies. Polymyositis, fasciitis, trichinosis, steroid atrophy, and acute alcohol myopathy may all have a significant pain component in addition to weakness. With rheumatoid arthritis and polymyalgia rheumatica there may be significant myalgias with little evidence of impaired muscle power. However, most patients with prominent myalgias in the absence of weakness turn out to have an endogenous depressive neurosis. Severeal acute denervating disorders may present significant muscle soreness and aching. In acute brachial neuritis

Table 1-6. Muscle Discomfort

	Cramps	Twitching (Fasciculations, Myokymia)	Myalgias	Stiffness
Muscle	hypothyroid myopathy disorders of muscle energy metabolism		myositis fasciitis trichinosis polymyalgia steroid myopathy ? MADA deficiency	myotonias
Nerve	peripheral neuropathy motor neuron disease Isaac's disease	peripheral neuropathy motor neuron disease Isaac's disease		Isaac's disease tetanus
Other	"benign" cramps drugs uremia	hyperthyroidism hyperparathyroidism "benign" fasciculations drugs		stiff-man syndrome spacticity rigidity apraxia

there are usually severe pains involving the shoulder(s), followed in a few days by proximal weakness. This disorder may be confused with an inflammatory myopathy in which case electrical studies (electromyography) are extremely valuable.   Diabetic amyotrophy may produce a similar symptom complex.

Muscle stiffness and/or slowness usually reflect upper motor neuron dysfunction. Such complaints are characteristic of patients with pyramidal tract spasticity, basal ganglia rigidity, or frontal lobe apraxia. However, myotonic disordera and hypothyroid myopathy may also be responsible. Such patients may relate that cold weather and immobility exacerbate their stiffness (a complaint often ascribed by the unwary examiner to "arthritis"). When stiffness is accompanied by the development of stone-hard, board-like muscles, the diagnosis of the stiff-man syndrome should be considered. This is an unusual disorder which begins with episodic tightness in the axial musculature. Over a period of months, it progresses to continuous muscle stiffness involving limbs, trunk, and neck. Excessive tonic innervation to intrafusal fibers of the muscle spindle appears to be the underlying pathophysiology. Excellent relief may be obtained with diazepam or baclofen (Whelan, 1980). Another unusual disorder in which stiffness may be the dominant symptom is the syndrome of continuous muscle fiber activity. Described by Isaacs in 1961, the disorder is characterized clinically by stiffness in limb musculature, muscle undulations (myokymia), hyperhydrosis, and focal muscle hypertrophy. Phenytoin or carbamazipine may provide effective relief of symptoms. Figure 1-2 summarizes much of what has been discussed above.

Organic Versus Functional Symptoms

Often it is difficult to determine on the basis of the history alone whether the patient's complaints are real or fictitious. However, with regard to some neuromuscular complaints, certain aspects of the patient's story may be revealing. Weakness that is vaguely described and that involves all muscle groups equally should raise suspicion as to its authenticity. Hysterics and malingerers seldom describe distinct motor problems (i.e., difficulty climbing stairs or unscrewing jar lids). Instead, every task is equally difficult to perform and lack of energy is frequently emphasized in their story.

Diplopia is another common symptom of organic neuromuscular disease frequently adopted by hysterics and malingerers. When evaluating this symptom, certain historical aspects are helpful in distinguishing true from feigned diplopia. One should always ask the patient if there are any maneuvers which ameliorate the double vision. With rare exceptions, organic diplopia disappears when one eye is closed or covered. Typically, hysterics relate that closing either eye has no effect on the double image. They may further betray their nonorganic condition by complaining of triplopia or quadriplopia.

Individuals with organic neuromuscular disease as well as hysterics may ex-

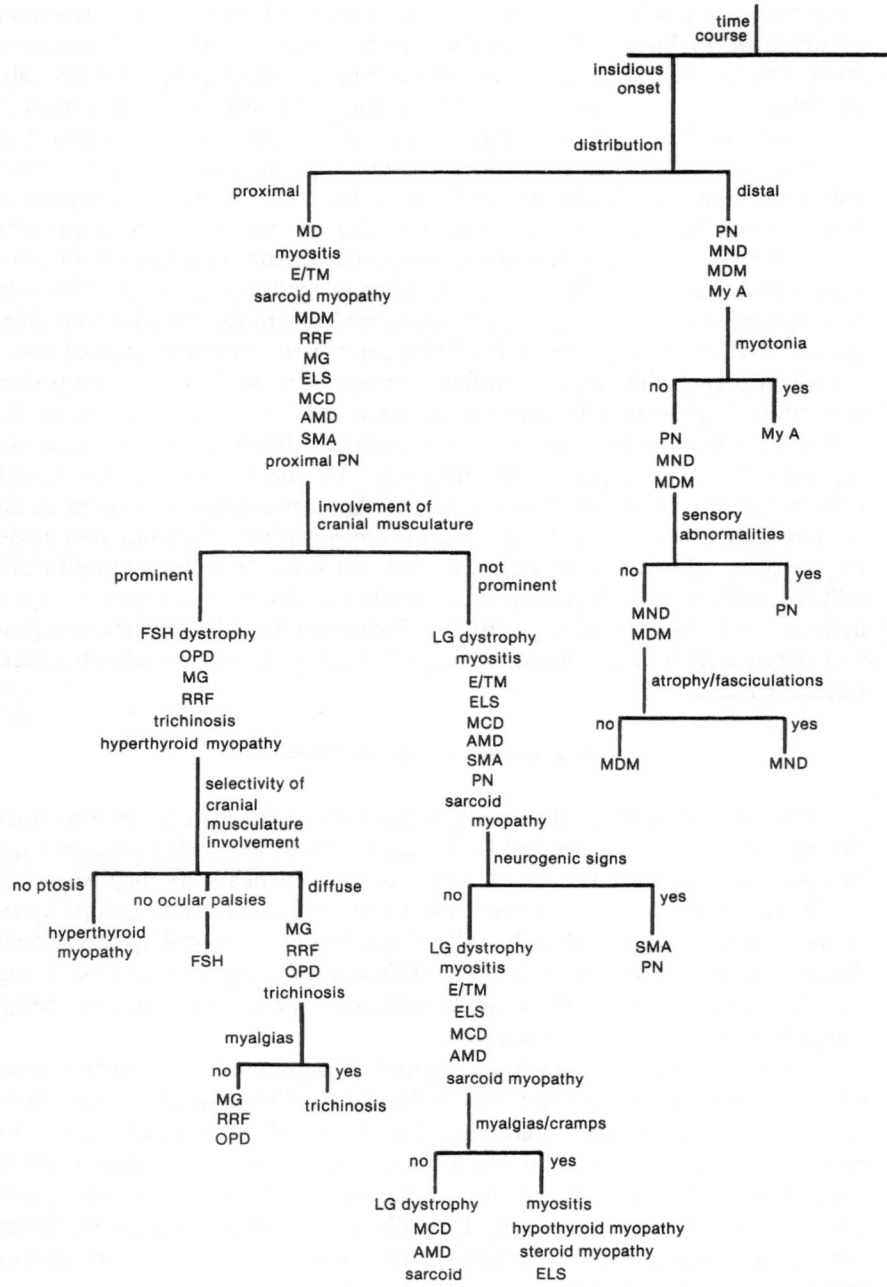

Figure 1.2. Summary flow chart. Symptom: symmetric weakness.

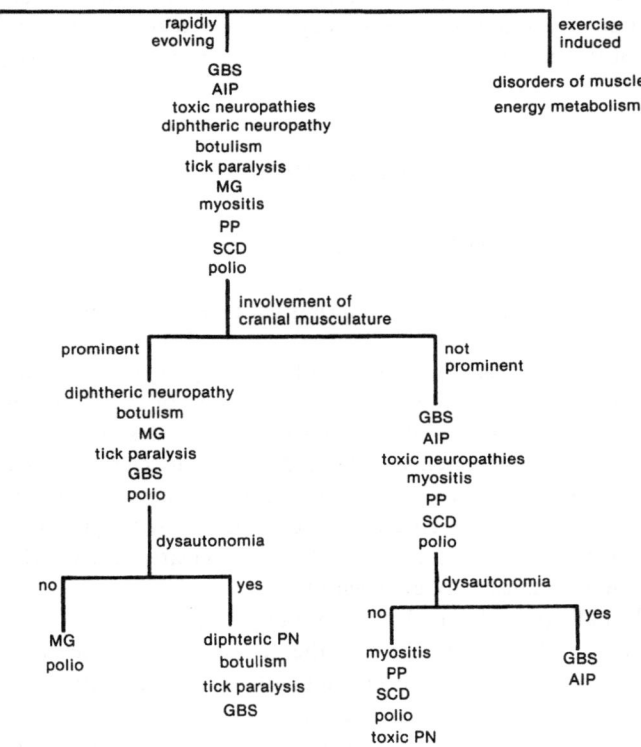

```
                    rapidly                                    exercise
                    evolving │                                 induced │

                       GBS
                       AIP                              disorders of muscle
                  toxic neuropathies                    energy metabolism
                 diphtheric neuropathy
                     botulism
                    tick paralysis
                       MG
                     myositis
                       PP
                      SCD
                      polio
                              │ involvement of
                                cranial musculature

        prominent │                              │ not
                                                   prominent

         diphtheric neuropathy
             botulism
               MG                            GBS
           tick paralysis                    AIP
             GBS                        toxic neuropathies
             polio                          myositis
                                              PP
                                             SCD
                                             polio
                    │ dysautonomia
                                                     │ dysautonomia
      no │                │ yes                no │              │ yes

        MG          diphteric PN           myositis          GBS
       polio          botulism                PP             AIP
                    tick paralysis           SCD
                       GBS                   polio
                                           toxic PN
```

KEY TO ABBREVIATIONS

AIP = acute intermittent porphyria
AMD = acid maltase deficiency
ELS = Eaton-Lambert syndrome
E/TM = endocrine/toxic myopathies
FSH = fascio scapulohumeral
GBS = Guillain-Barre syndrome
LG = limb-girdle
MCD = muscle carnitine deficiency
MD = muscular dystrophy
MDM = morphologically distinct myopathies
MG = myasthenia gravis
MyA = myotonic atrophy
OPD = oculopharyngeal dystrophy
PN = peripheral neuropathy
PP = periodic paralysis
RRF = ragged-red fiber disease
SCD = systemic carnitine deficiency
SMA = spinal muscular atrophy

perience difficult and painful swallowing. Patients with functional dysphagia commonly describe the sensation of food sticking in the back of the throat. This hysterical sensation may last for hours or days. Nasal regurgitation and aspiration, hallmarks of organic dysphagia, are seldom reported by such individuals.

SIGNS OF NEUROMUSCULAR DISEASE

Physical Examination

Examination of the neuromuscular system begins with a rapid yet thorough general inspection of the patient.

If distal weakness is the major complaint, looking for premature frontal balding and testicular atrophy suggestive of myotonic atrophy, or for bony abnormalities (i.e., pes cavus), hallmarks of hereditary neuropathies, is useful. Skeletal deformities including high arched palate, dental malocclusions, and clubfoot are also commonly found in association with the morphologically distinct myopathies including central core and rod disease. With proximal weakness, inspecting the skin for the changes of dermatomyositis, sarcoidosis, chronic steroid use, or alcohol abuse may be rewarding.

Changes in muscle bulk (atrophy and hypertrophy), if present, may be a helpful finding. When atrophy occurs early in the course of neuromuscular weakness, it generally signifies axonal neurogenic disease. In contrast with most myopathies, neuromuscular junction disorders, and demyelinating neuropathies, there is little atrophy in the initial stages of this disease. Focal muscle hypertrophy is characteristic of certain myopathies including several of the dystrophies, while in hypothyroid myopathy (Hoffman's syndrome) and myotonia congenita there is generalized muscle enlargement. Muscles may also appear enlarged when they are infiltrated with parasitis (i.e., cysticercosis), amyloid deposits (Ringel et al, 1982), or granulomas (sarcoidosis). In addition, some neuropathies may also produce focal muscle hypertrophy (i.e., spinal muscular atrophies and Isaacs' disease).

The presence of spontaneous muscle twitches should be carefully noted. Visible muscle twitches are either fasciculations or myokymia ("live flesh"). Fibrillations are too small to be seen except perhaps in the tongue.

Fasciculations are fine, rapid, flickering movements that appear with contraction of a bundle of fibers from a single motor unit. They are best seen in superficial muscles and may be induced by tapping or cooling the muscle. Prominent fasciculations occur with anterior horn cell disease, but may also be seen with axonal neuropathies, radiculopathies, tetany, thyrotoxicosis, and anticholinesterase medications. Spontaneous, fine, worm-like muscle undulations (myokymia) also occur with primary neurogenic diseases and are especially prominent in the syndrome of continuous muscle fiber activity (Isaacs, 1961).

Electrically, myokymia consists of repetitive trains of normal action potentials producing brief tetanic contractions of muscle fibers of a motor unit.

After inspection, the muscles should be palpated. Exquisitely tender muscles may occur with inflammatory muscle diseases, fasciitis, polymyalgia rheumatica, steroid myopathy, and acute alcohol myopathy. If subcutaneous nodules are present, entities such as sarcoidosis, cysticercosis, and calcinosis (as seen in dermatomyositis) should be considered. The peripheral nerves should also be quickly assessed as to their size. Enlarged nerves are characteristically seen in leprosy, the hereditary motor/sensory neuropathies (i.e., Charcot-Marie-Tooth, Dejerine-Sottas and Refsum's disease), and chronic recurrent inflammatory polyneuropathies.

After inspection and palpation, attention should be turned to the muscles of the cranial nerves with special attention to the lid elevators, ocular, facial, pharyngeal, and neck muscles. Weakness of the lid elevators results in lids which partially cover the pupillary aperture. An increase in the number of forehead creases and an ipsilateral elevated eyebrow are common accompaniments of ptosis, and reflect the patient's attempt to overcome the drooping of the lids by contracting the frontalis muscles. The patient with subtle ptosis may also maintain the head in a mildly hyperextended position in order to see straight ahead. Ptosis may occur with lesions of the sympathetic nerves (producing Horner's syndrome) or with third nerve palsies. However, in these conditions, there are accompanying pupillary abnormalities (i.e., meiosis with the former condition and mydriasis with the latter). Ptosis that alternates from side to side is virtually pathognomonic of myasthenia gravis.

One of the most frequent causes of ptosis especially in the elderly is the levator dehisence-disinsertion syndrome (Thompson et al, 1982). In this condition, the ptosis is caused by a structural abnormality in the aponeurosis of the levator palpebrae muscle. Unlike patients with ptosis secondary to neuromuscular disease, these patients are able to voluntarily elevate the lid more than 12 mm.

Motility of the extraocular muscles can be rapidly assessed by having the patient follow a target in the cardinal fields of gaze and noting any deficits. More subtle paresis can be elicited by the red glass or alternate cover tests (Glaser, 1978). Prominent ptosis and ophthalmoplegia typically occur with myasthenia gravis, botulism, "ragged-red" fiber disease, as well as with some neuropathies (i.e., diphtheric neuropathy). Ptosis without major disturbances in ocular motility is characteristic of myotonic atrophy and oculopharyngeal dystrophy, whereas ophthalmoparesis without ptosis occurs in Graves' ophthalmopathy (exophthalmic ophthalmoplegia). Of course central nervous system disorders may also impair ocular motility. However, these can usually be eliminated by a careful neurologic examination. Asymmetry of ptosis or ophthalmoplegia is common in neuromuscular diseases and should not dissuade you from the diagnosis (see Table 1-3).

Assessment of strength in the facial muscles can be made by having the patient wrinkle his forehead, close his eyes, smile, and keep the cheeks puffed with air. Patients with weakness of the orbicularis oculi are unable to bury the eyelashes when asked to squeeze their eyes forcefully shut. When attempting to smile, patients with facial weakness produce an unpleasant snarl which is often a source of embarassment. Pursing the lips or maintaining the cheeks puffed with air is difficult. Typically, patients with myotonic atrophy, facioscapulohumeral dystrophy, morphologically distinct myopathies, myasthenia gravis, and botulism have significant facial paresis. It is not unusual, however, for peripheral nerve disorders (i.e., Guillain-Barré syndrome and sarcoidosis) and anterior horn cell diseases also to involve these structures. However, when weakness of the orbicularis oculi is added to ocular palsies and ptosis, it nearly always signals a myopathic process.

Weakness of the palatal, labial, or lingual muscles may produce dysarthic speech. Typically, patients with labial weakness will have problems articulating "M," "B," and "P," whereas "L" and "T" are more problematic with lingual dysarthria. Guttural sounds ("NK" and "NG") are affected when there is impaired palatal function. Certain test phrases such as "Methodist Episcopal" and "eleven benevolent elephants" are helpful in accentuating these articulation problems. In contrast, with impaired laryngeal function, there is hoarseness and dysphonia. Dysarthria and/or dysphonia are frequent manifestations of myotonic atrophy, oculopharyngeal muscular dystrophy, myositis, myasthenia gravis, and botulism. Neurogenic diseases including Guillain-Barré syndrome, diphtheric neuropathy, and anterior horn cell disease may also have prominent dysarthria and/or dysphonia. However, in these latter disorders, other signs of neurogenic disease including changes in the activity of the gag reflex, fasciculations, and atrophy of the tongue, should be evident.

In contrast, disordered cranial nerve function is unusual in the Eaton-Lambert syndrome, periodic paralysis, Duchenne-type muscular dystrophy, and steroid and alcohol myopathy (see Table 1-4).

The examination continues with the assessment of limb and girdle strength. During this part of the examination, it is important to determine the topography of the limb weakness (i.e., symmetric versus localized, proximal versus distal). Most primary muscle disorders produce symmetric weakness. Focal loss of strength limited to one extremity or one side of the body suggests neuronal disease (i.e., radiculopathy, neuropathy, or central nervous system dysfunction). Weakness in a proximal distribution suggests primary muscle or junction disease whereas distal weakness is more commonly seen in neurogenic disorders. However, as discussed previously, there are numerous exceptions to this generalization (see Tables 1-1 and 4-1).

Careful observation of the patient prior to formal muscle testing is helpful and will provide clues as to the distribution of the weakness. Patients with shoulder girdle weakness may demonstrate abnormalities of posture and gait. Such individuals may walk with the backs of their hands facing forward rather than to the side. This is due to abnormal rotation of the shoulders. The arms may also appear to be hanging limply when the patient is standing. In addition, winging of the scapula may be evidence indicative of weakness of the serratus anterior, rhomboids, or trapezius muscles. Loss of power in the hip abductors and other proximal lower extremity muscles produces a waddling, lordotic gait. The shoulders may be thrown back when the patient is walking in order to shift the center of gravity posteriorly so that the bony structures of the hips assume more of a weight-bearing function. In addition, patients with hip girdle weakness may perform a characteristic series of maneuvers when attempting to arise from the floor (Gowers' sign). When instructed to stand from a prone position the patient will initially tuck the knees under the trunk. The knees are then extended so that the patient is now supported on all fours with the hips arched high off the ground. The patient then places the hands on the knees and "walks" them up the thighs while simultaneously extending the trunk to achieve the desired erect posture.

Distal weakness of the upper extremities may be suspected when there are changes in the posture of the hands. Normally the thumb is at a right angle to the remaining fingers. When the thumb is on the same plane, it usually reflects loss of strength in some of the intrinsic hand musculature. With distal weakness of the lower limbs involving the ankle dorsiflexors, the patient will have a characteristic gait. As the patient walks, the knees are lifted higher than normal and the foot slaps down onto the floor. Heel walking is impossible. With loss of strength in the plantar flexors, the patient is unable to hop or ride up on toes, one foot at a time.

After the patient's gait, posture, and performance of these simple maneuvers have been observed, formal muscle testing should be performed. The Medical Research Council of Great Britain recognizes five grades of muscle strength:

0. No contraction
1. Flicker or trace of contraction
2. Active joint movement when gravity is eliminated
3. Active joint movement against gravity
4. Active joint movement against gravity and resistance
5. Normal power

This system is useful and serves as a rough quantitative measure of muscle power.

The muscle stretch reflexes are next evaluated, and traditionally the biceps, triceps, brachioradialis, quadriceps and achilles reflexes are tested. These should be recorded as either absent, diminshed, normal, or hyperactive. In most myopathies, the reflexes are preserved until late in the illness. In contrast, patients with large fiber neuropathies (those that involve the Aα or Aγ efferent or Iα afferent nerve fibers) often lose their reflexes prior to the development of other symptoms or signs. However, with small fiber neuropathies (i.e., amyloid neuropathy), there is preservation of the muscle stretch reflexes. With the reflex hammer still in hand, the examiner should tap the thenar eminences and forearm extensor surfaces in search of myotonia and/or myoedema. Myotonia is characteristic of myotonic atrophy, myotonia congenita, paramyotonia, and some of the periodic paralyses. Myoedema is seen with hypothyroid myopathy. The cerebellar and sensory systems are then evaluated to uncover auxilliary clues of neuromuscular syndromes (i.e., the ataxia of "ragged-red" fiber disease and the sensory loss ofperipheral neuropathies).

Organic Versus Functional Signs

Distinguishing true weakness from malingering is often not an easy task, even for the experienced examiner. However, organic weakness usually has characteristic qualities. The examiner can overcome the patient's best effort to resist him, and the resistance which the muscle displays is uniform throughout the range of movement. With nonorganic weakness, the resistance encountered by the examiner varies with the examiner's effort, and the "giving way" phenomenon is apparent. (The initial resistance offered is strong; then suddenly all power is lost.) Alternately, the patient may have small contractions followed by periods of relaxation. This results in a repetitive catch and give phenomenon.

A useful maneuver in evaluating a patient with "suspect" weakness is to palpate the antagonist muscle (i.e., triceps) while the agonist (i.e., biceps) is being tested. If one feels contraction in the triceps when the patient is asked to flex the elbow, all is not "kosher."

Finally, a "suspicious" patient should be closely observed (when he is unaware of scrutiny) to see if he makes any movements which he denies being able to perform upon command.

SUMMARY

Analysis of the patient's complaints in combination with a thorough physical examination enables the physician to derive a reasonable list of possible diagnoses. For further clarification of the problem, however, appropriate laboratory studies and procedures may be necessary. These are discussed in detail in Chapter 2.

CHAPTER 2

Laboratory Aids for Diagnosing Neuromuscular Diseases

BASIC ANATOMY AND PHYSIOLOGY OF THE MOTOR UNIT

Frequently, laboratory studies are necessary to arrive at the specific cause of a neuromuscular problem. Electrodiagnostic studies and microscopic examination of muscle tissue are particularly essential for this purpose. A basic knowledge of neuromuscular anatomy and physiology is helpful for the best use of these tests.

The motor unit is the functional unit of the neuromuscular system. It is made up of a motor neuron whose cell body lies within the anterior horn of the spinal cord, its single axon which leaves the cord in the ventral root, and the muscle fibers which it innervates. The points of "contact" between the terminal twigs of the motor neuron and the muscle fibers are called the neuromuscular junctions.

Motor units vary in size depending on the individual muscle. For example, in the lumbrical muscles of the hand, there are an estimated 100 fibers per motor unit, while in the gastrocnemius, almost 2,000 muscle fibers are innervated by a single sacral anterior horn cell.

Because each muscle fiber is embryologically derived from the fusion of many myoblasts, mature fibers contain hundreds of nuclei which are normally subsarcolemmal in location. The cytoplasm (sarcoplasm) contains the usual types of inclusions including mitochondria and sarcoplasmic reticulum (SR). Surrounding the fiber is a cell membrane (sarcolemma) from which membranous invaginations originate. These structures, called T tubules, run perpendicular to the sarcoplasmic reticulum and at regular intervals contact dilations of the SR (cisternae) to form a triad (see Figure 2-1).

Unique to the muscle fiber are structures called myofibrils that under the electron microscope are shown to be made up of hundreds of units called sarco-

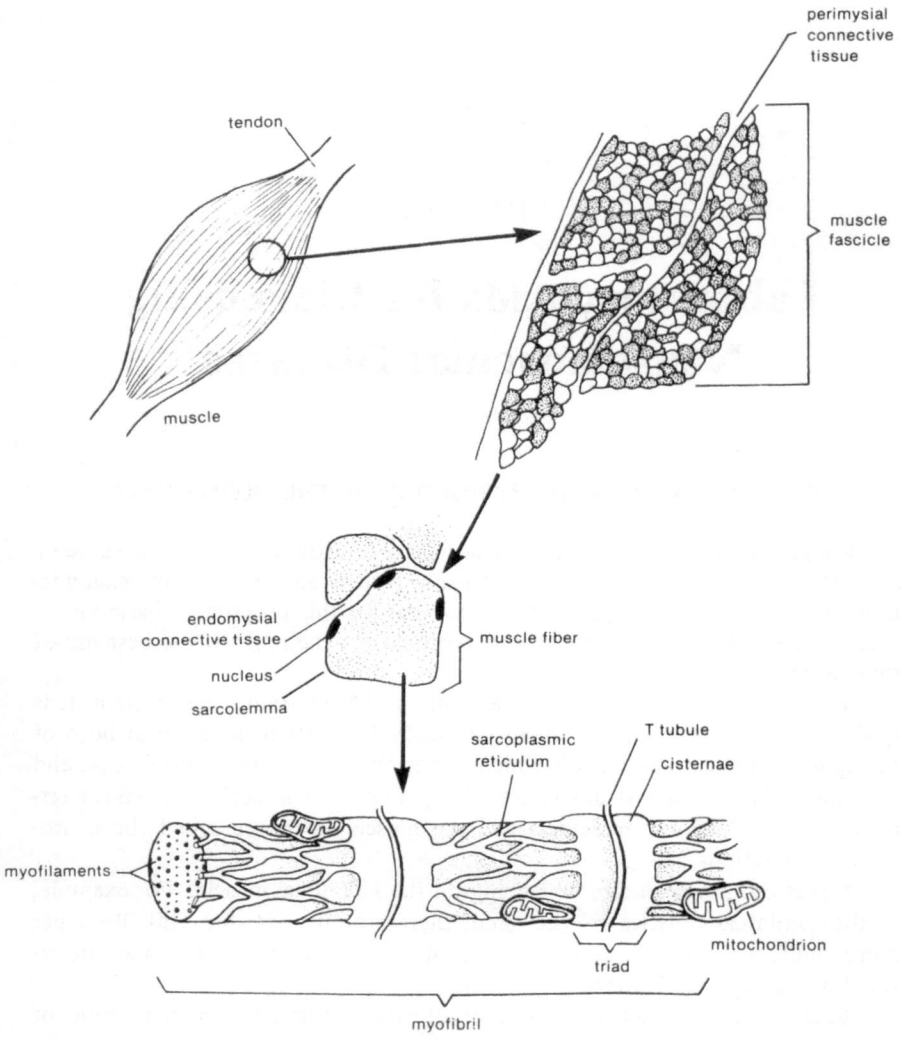

Figure 2-1.   Muscle anatomy.

meres (see Figure 2-2). Within these sarcomeres are the thin and thick myofilaments. Thin myofilaments are composed of three separate proteins: actin, tropomyosin, and troponin. Myosin is the chief constituent of the thick filaments. It
has ATP-ase (enzyme) activity and actin-binding sites.

The interdigitating arrangement of the myofilaments produces the characteristic striated appearance of skeletal muscle. The dark A band corresponds to
the region of overlap of the thin and thick filaments. In the midsection is a less
dense strip, the H zone, where only thick filaments are present. The light areas
or I bands contain only thin filaments. The dense Z lines limit the sarcomere.
Triads are located at the A-I junctions.

In general, the most widely accepted theory of muscle contraction is the
sliding filament hypothesis (Huxley and Hanson, 1954). According to this
theory, the thin and thick filaments slide past each other during a contraction,
thereby shortening the sarcomere and the muscle fiber. The lengths of the filaments themselves do not change. When the nerve action potential arrives at the
motor nerve terminal, it induces the release of acetylcholine (the chemical
transmitter of the neuromuscular junction). After diffusing across the synaptic
cleft, the acetylcholine interacts with specific receptors located on the muscle
membrane. This interaction changes the characteristics of the muscle membrane
so that it now exhibits increased permeability to sodium ions. Influxing sodium
ions depolarize the muscle membrane to the threshold whereby a muscle action
potential is generated (see Chapter 3 for further details regarding neuromuscular
transmission). The muscle action potential is then propagated along the sarcolemma and is conveyed into the fiber's interior via the T tubules. At the region
of the triad, the wave of depolarization spreads to the SR and initiates the release of Ca^{++} from the cisternae. The Ca^{++} binds to troponin depressing its in-
hibitory effect on actin-myosin cross bridge formation. Actin and myosin are
now free to interact and form bonds. The formation and cleavage of such cross
bridges produce active movement of the filaments along their lengths. Energy
in the form of ATP is required for this process. Relaxation involves the re-uptake of Ca^{++} by the SR. Unbound troponin now inhibits the actin-myosin interaction so that cross bridges can no longer be formed, and the muscle returns to
its resting length. Further details on the mechanism of muscle contraction are
provided by Huxley (1969).

ELECTRODIAGNOSTIC TESTING

The clinician who is confronted with a neuromuscular problem but is unde-
cided after physical examination as to where the pathology lies (i.e., anterior
horn cell, peripheral nerve, neuromuscular junction or muscle) should begin the
investigation with an electroneuromyogram (ENMG).

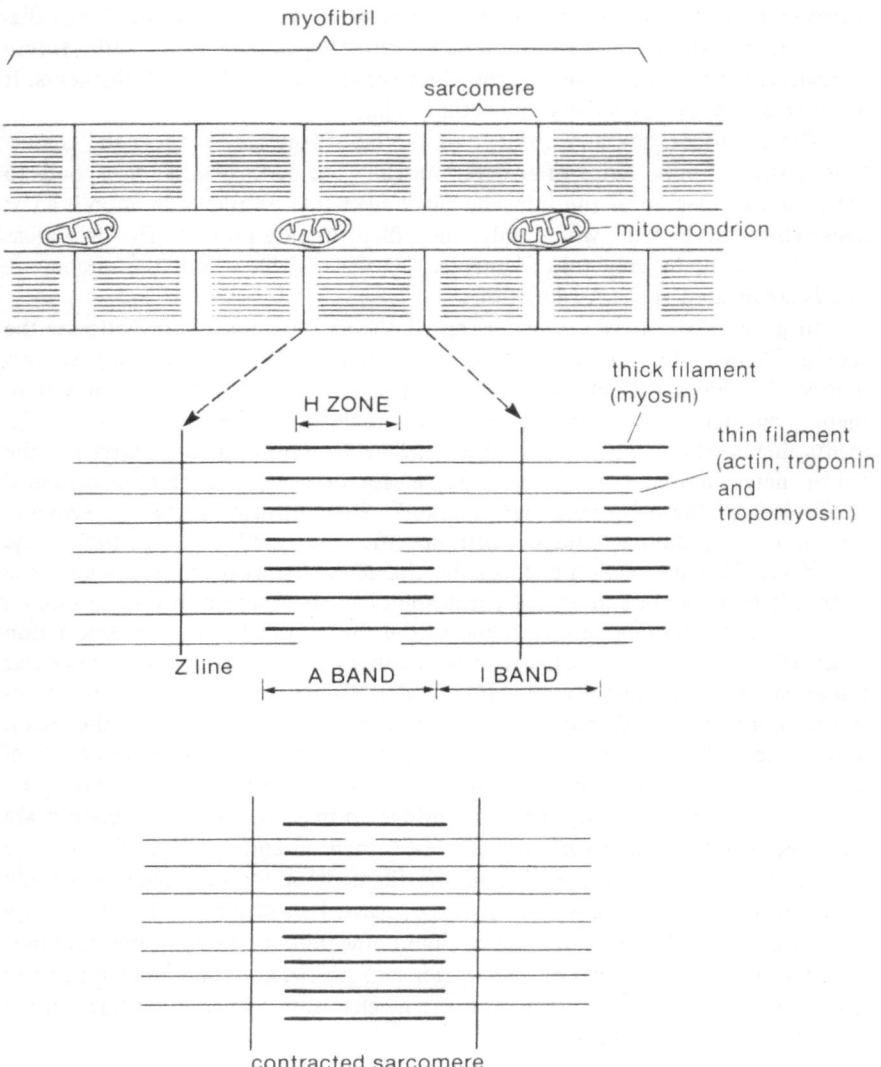

Figure 2-2. The sarcomere.

Electrodiagnostic testing is a useful supplement to the clinical neuromuscular examination. The basic electrical examination (ENMG) consists of two parts: (1) measurement of nerve conduction velocities, and (2) needle electromyography. Nerve conduction studies (motor and sensory) help to differentiate neurogenic from myopathic diseases. Electromyography allows one to sample numerous muscles which is important considering the patchy involvement of some disease processes, and it can also help localize the disease process to one or more components of the neuromuscular system, thereby providing clues as to etiology.

Repetitive nerve stimulation studies are not part of the routine ENMG but are included when one suspects a disorder of neuromuscular transmission (i.e., myasthenia gravis, Eaton-Lambert syndrome and botulism). This is discussed further in Chapter 3.

Nerve Conduction Velocities

Determining conduction velocities involves stimulating the nerve at one or more points and recording the response either at the muscle (for motor nerve conduction studies) or at some distance along the nerve from the overlying skin (for sensory nerve conduction rates). In the extremities, the median, ulnar, radial, peroneal, and posterior tibial nerves are most accessible to such measurements. The compound motor action potential (CMAP) and sensory nerve action potental (SNAP) have certain measureable parameters including (see Figure 2-3):

1. Latency, which is defined as the time between the shock artifact and the onset of the evoked response. It reflects conduction in the fastest fibers.
2. Amplitude, which correlates with the number of fibers conducting and the degree of asynchrony. A low amplitude implies loss of axons.
3. Duration, which is the temporal dispersion of the response and depends on the difference in the conduction velocities between the fastest and slowest fibers.

The conduction velocity is calculated by determining the difference in the latencies between two points of stimulation along a single nerve and dividing this number into the distance between these same two points (see Figure 2-4). While minimal degrees of slowing (i.e., velocities reduced by less than thirty percent of normal) can be seen with axonal disorders, decreased nerve conduction velocities usually indicate disease of the peripheral nerve myelin. Nerve conduction velocities are normal with primary myopathic and junctional disorders.

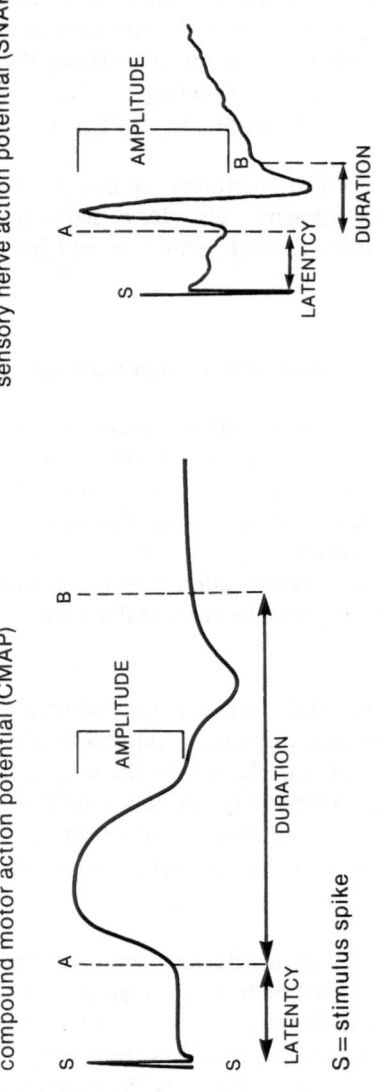

Figure 2.3. Evoked response.

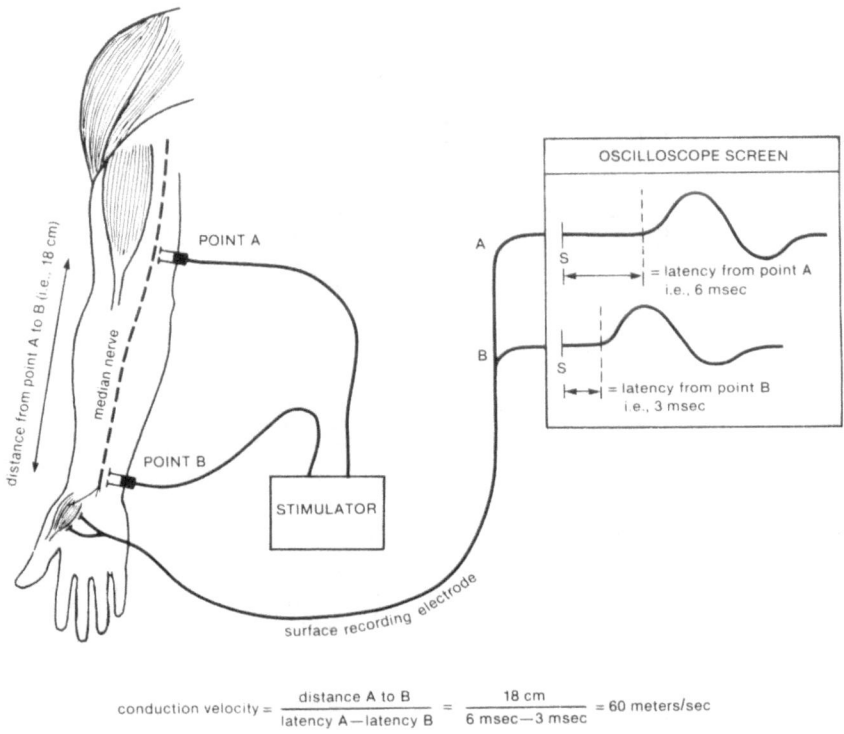

$$\text{conduction velocity} = \frac{\text{distance A to B}}{\text{latency A} - \text{latency B}} = \frac{18 \text{ cm}}{6 \text{ msec} - 3 \text{ msec}} = 60 \text{ meters/sec}$$

Figure 2-4. Motor nerve conduction velocity measurement.

Electromyography

Needle electromyography involves recording electrical activity from muscle at rest and with attempted volitional activity. Normal resting muscle is electrically silent except for a brief burst of potentials that occur with insertion of the needle. When the EMG needle is moved briskly in the muscle, injury potentials are produced. These potentials called "positive sharp waves" are easily recognized by their initial sharp positivity (downward deflection) followed by a long duration negative (upward) component (see Table 2-1). In normal muscle, these potentials disappear abruptly when needle movement ceases. This is what is meant by normal insertional activity. Denervated muscle and myotonic muscle are characterized by prolonged insertional activity: that is, there are runs of positive sharp waves even after the EMG needle is no longer moving. End stage

Table 2-1. EMG Potentials

	Amplitude	Duration	Frequency	Rhythm	Form	Sound
end plate noise	<50 μv	1-3 msec	20-25/sec	irreg	monophasic	seashell murmur
end plate spike	20-200 μv	3-5 msec	up to 50/sec	irreg	diphasic	cracking
positive sharp wave	50-200 μv	10-30 msec	10/sec	irreg/reg	diphasic	dull pop
fibrillation	20-200 μv	1-5 sec	2-20/sec	reg	diphasic	rain on the roof
simple fasciculation	300-5000 μv	3-16 msec	1-50/min	ireg	bi, triphasic	dull pop
complex fasciculations	>5000 μv	>16 msec	1-50/min	irreg	polyphasic	dull pop
motor unit potential	300-5000 μv	3-16 msec	5-50/sec	reg	bi, triphasic	–
"giant" motor unit potential	>5000 μv	>16 msec	5-50/sec	reg	polyphasic	–
"BSAPP"	<300 μv	<3 msec	5-50/sec	reg	polyphasic	–

Table 2-2. Diseases with Fibrillations

Neurogenic	Myopathic	Other
motor neuron disease	inflammatory myopathies (myositis trichinosis)	hypo/hyperkalemia
axonal neuropathies	dystrophies	muscle trauma
radiculopathies	myotonic atrophy "congenital/myopathies" hyperkalemic periodic paralysis acid maltase deficiency	

muscle (i.e., muscle that has been extensively replaced by fat and connective tissue) and muscles examined *during* an acute episode of periodic paralysis have diminished insertional activity.

When probing the muscle, the needle may inadvertently contact a neuromuscular junction. One may record end plate noise, end plate spikes, and positive sharp waves from this region (see Table 2-1). End plate noise is a series of high frequency, negative (upward deflection) discharges of low amplitude. Over the loudspeaker, these discharges produce a seashell murmur. They probably represent needle recordings of miniature end plate potentials induced by the needle mechanically stimulating acetylcholine (ACh) release. If enough ACh is liberated, muscle action potentials are generated and potentials called end plate spikes appear. These discharges have the same amplitude and duration as fibrillations, but a different configuration and firing pattern. If the needle electrode is advanced slightly so that it is now recording from an injured fiber, positive sharp waves will appear. Remember, end plate noise and end plate spikes followed by positive sharp waves are found in normal muscle.

Abnormal spontaneous discharges include fibrillations, fasciculations, myotonia, neuromyotonia, myokymia, and bizarre repetitive potentials.

Fibrillation potentials are spontaneous discharges from individual muscle fibers. They are easily recognized by their small amplitude and biphasic configuration (initial downward deflection followed by an upward phase). While commonly seen with neurogenic (axonal) diseases, fibrillations are not synonymous with denervation. They are also prominent in some of the myopathies, including polymyositis, trichinosis and facioscapulohumeral dystrophy (see Table 2-2).

Fasciculations are the action potentials of a group of fiber innervated by a common anterior horn cell. They have the same amplitude and duration as a voluntary motor unit potential but are distinguished by their slow, irregular firing pattern. Fasciculation potentials may occur in normal individuals ("benign" or "simple" fasciculations) as well as in neuromuscular diseases (see

Table 2-3.   Disease with Fasciculations

Neurogenic	Other
motor neuron disease	benign fasciculations
axonal neuropathies	thyrotoxicosis
radiculopathies	hyperparathyroidism
Jakob-Creutzfeldt	drugs
	tetany

Table 2-3). "Complex" fasciculations tend to be larger in amplitude, polyphasic, and to fire at a somewhat slower frequency. These are generally seen in motor neuron disease.

High frequency discharges consisting of extended trains of potentials with varying frequency and amplitude are characteristic of the myotonias (see Table 2-4).

Such potentials may take one of two forms depending on the relationship of the recording electrode to the muscle fiber. When initiated by needle insertion, these potentials have the configuration of positive sharp waves. Both amplitude and frequency may increase or decrease as the discharge continues. Myotonia induced by voluntary activity appears as brief spike potentials resembling fibrillations. Over the loudspeaker they produce a "dive bomber" sound.

Other abnormal spontaneous potentials, including myokymia, neuromyotonia, and bizarre high frequency potentials, are seen in a variety of neuromuscular diseases. Further details regarding these discharges are beyond the scope of this book.

After the muscle at rest is studied, the needle is left in place and the patient is asked to contract the muscle voluntarily. When an anterior horn cell is activated, an action potential travels down its axon and terminal nerve fibers to produce an almost synchronous depolarization of muscle fibers that it innervates. The summated potential generated by these fibers is the motor unit potential (MUP). Actually, the full complement of muscle fibers innervated by

Table 2-4.   Diseases with Myotonia

myotonic atrophy
myotonia congenita
paramyotonia
hyperkalemic periodic paralysis
acid maltase deficiency
polymyositis
drugs (diazocholesterol)
hypothyroidism

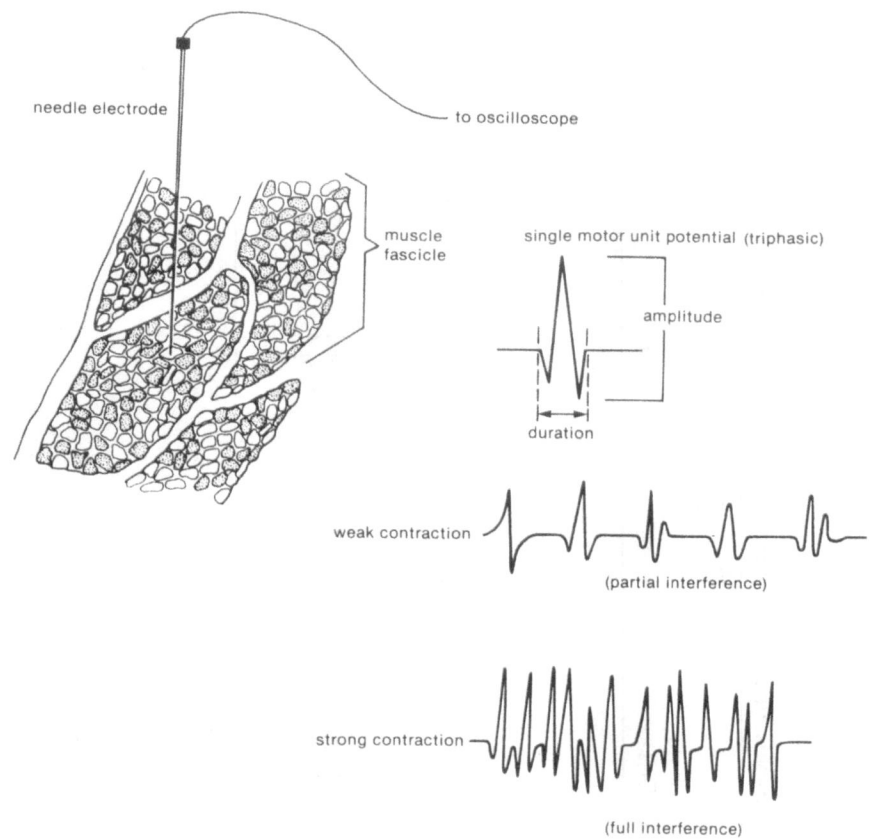

Figure 2-5. The normal EMG.

one anterior horn cell lies in an area that exceeds the effective pickup zone of the needle, so what is called the MUP is really only a fraction of the whole. A motor unit potential has characteristic amplitude, duration, and contour (see Table 2-1). Its amplitude is a function of the number of activated muscle fibers that lie close to the needle. Its duration reflects the degree of synchrony of firing between the fibers. Normally, the MUP has two to four phases but in certain disease states, may be polyphasic (i.e., greater than four phases).

With a weak contraction, one or two MUP's are observed on the oscilloscope. With increased effort, the rate of discharge increases and additional motor units are recruited. This produces a recording of many potentials firing

Table 2-5. Electromyographic Findings in Neurogenic and Myopathic Diseases

	Anterior Horn Cell Disease	Peripheral Neuropathy		Myopathy
		Demyelinative	Axonal	
nerve conduction studies				
amplitudes of evoked responses		N	↓	N
conduction velocities	N, or mildly ↓	↓↓	N, or mildly ↓	N
EMG				
insertional activity	↑	N	↑	N, ↑(in myotonias) ↓ (end stage muscle)
spontaneous potentials				
fibrillations	++	—	++	— or +
fasciculations	+++	—	+	—
voluntary motor units				
amplitude	↑↑	N	N or ↑	↓
duration	↑↑	N	N or ↑	↓
polyphasic potentials	+	—	+	+
recruitment	↓↓	N	↓	↑

↑ = increased
↓ = decreased
+ = present
N = normal

asynchronously. As greater tension develops, many motor units firing at high frequency interfere with one another so that single potentials can no longer be discriminated. This results in a complete interference pattern and in normal muscle it is clearly observed during strong contractions (see Figure 2-5).

Myopathic Versus Neurogenic Changes

Since the number of functioning fibers per motor unit is reduced in myopathies and junctional disorders, it is not surprising that the motor unit potentials in these diseases are small in amplitude, short in duration, and polyphasic. Because individual motor units are small, a given range of movement or tension requires a greater firing rate and recruitment of motor units. Thus a total interference pattern is seen at a phase of activity far lower than expected. The acronym BSAPP (brief in duration, small in amplitude, abundant for the effort called on to produce, polyphasic potentials) is often used to describe this pattern. Sometimes the BSAPP pattern is erroneously referred to as the "myopathic pattern." This should be avoided because it has been shown that such changes are not specific of a primary myopathic process (Engel, 1975) (i.e., BSAPPs may be seen in early reinnervation after nerve damage).

Electrodiagnostic findings in neurogenic disease vary with the site of pathology and the duration of the process (see Table 2-5). Demyelinative peripheral neuropathies are characterized electrically by slow nerve conduction velocities and a normal EMG. The pattern of slowing may provide clues as to the etiology (Lewis and Sumner 1982). Familial demyelinative neuropathies (i.e., Charcot-Marie-Tooth disease) tend to produce uniform slowing, whereas with the acquired varieties (i.e., diabetes and Guillain-Barré syndrome) the pattern is one of multifocal slowing.

With axonal neuropathies (i.e., toxic neuropathies) the conductions are normal (or *mildly* slowed) but the amplitudes of the evoked responses are low. Increased insertional activity, abnormal spontaneous discharges, and polyphasic voluntary potentials are present. Anterior horn cell diseases produce similar changes except that fasciculations are more prominent and the voluntary potentials tend to be extremely large in amplitude and long in duration (giant potentials). Giant potentials indicate that reinnervation has occurred by the process of collateral sprouting of surviving axonal twigs and imply a chronic process.

With moderate degrees of axonal pathology, there may be a reduction in the number of motor units so that a partial interference pattern is seen with maximal effort. In severe disease, a single motor unit interference pattern is observed. (Single motor unit potentials are seen separated by considerable lengths of flat base line even with maximal contraction of the muscle.) Such a pattern is characteristic of chronic motor neuron disease.

Table 2-6. Muscle Histology and Histochemistry

Stain	Myopathic Changes		Neuropathic Changes	
	Non-Specific	Specific	Deinnervation	Reinnervation
modified Gomori trichrome	basophilic fibers increased endo-mysial connective tissue	inflammatory infiltrates (myositis) "ragged-red" fibers rods	small angulated fibers	
ATPase		perifascicular atrophy (myositis)		type grouping
NADH-TR	cytoarchitectural changes	cores	target fibers dark angular fibers	target fibers type grouping
alkaline phosphatase	"regen-degen" fibers	positive staining of the connective tissue (myositis)		
esterase		macrophages (myositis)	small dark angular fibers	

More detailed information concerning electrodiagnostic studies are provided in the works by Goodgold and Eberstein, and Liveson and Spielholtz.

In conclusion, with the aid of electrical studies the clinician should be able to localize the disease process to the anterior horn cell, peripheral nerve, neuromuscular junction, or muscle. However, electrical studies while capable of defining the site of the lesion, seldom identify the specific disease process. For this purpose biopsy and histologic examination of nerve and muscle tissue are often needed.

MUSCLE HISTOLOGY AND HISTOCHEMISTRY

Muscle biopsy for the purpose of studying muscle histology and histochemistry may be necessary for the proper diagnosis of neuromuscular problems.

When selecting a muscle for biopsy, it is best to choose one that is, by clinical examination, partially involved by the disease process (i.e., one that is mildly atrophic with strength in the 3-4/5 range). A muscle that is severely atrophic and functionless probably will not yield diagnostic tissue. Every specimen of "end stage muscle" looks alike whether it is the victim of neurogenic or myopathic disease. A second consideration when choosing a muscle for biopsy is its surgical accessibility. In the upper extremities, the biceps or deltoid muscles are technically easy to sample, while in the lower limbs, the vastus lateralis is a good choice. Finally, a muscle that has been studied with EMG needles should not be chosen for biopsy. Needle artifact has accounted for many cases of "focal myositis."

Because many centers do a limited number of muscle stains, the physician in charge may be called upon to request special additional stains when indicated. Therefore it is important to have a working knowledge of the available stains and their clinical applicability. This is summarized in Tables 2-6 and 2-7 and discussed in the pages that follow.

Histology

For the investigation of neuromuscular diseases, both histologic and histochemical examination of muscle tissue are essential. Common histologic stains include hematoxylin and eosin (H & E) and the modified Gomori Trichrome (Engel and Cunningham, 1963). With the modified Gomori Trichrome (which in the author's opinion is superior to the H & E stain), the muscle fibers stain a greenish-blue color, the collagen a lighter but clearly distinguishable green color, and the nuclei red. The myelin of the nerve twigs stains red and the axons are bluish. The stain accentuates "ragged-red" fibers (see Figure 9-12) and rods (see Figure 5-5), and is excellent for demonstrating inflammatory infiltrates and

Table 2-7.   Essential Stains for Diagnosing Specific Myopathies

Suspected Myopathy	Stains Best Demonstrating Pathology
dystrophy	modified Gomori Trichrome alkaline phosphatase
polymyositis	modified Gomori Trichrome alkaline phosphatase esterase
endocrine myopathies	modified Gomori Trichrome ATP-ase
toxic myopathies	modified Gomori Trichrome ATP-ase
central core disease	NADH-TR
rod disease	modified Gomori Trichrome
type I fiber hypotrophy	modified Gomori Trichrome ATP-ase
"ragged-red" fiber disease	modified Gomori Trichrome
myotonic atrophy	modified Gomori Trichrome ATP-ase
periodic paralysis	modified Gomori Trichrome NADH-TR
disorders of muscle CHO/lipid metabolism	modified Gomori Trichrome myophosphorylase stain glycogen stain oil red O
myoadenylate deaminase deficiency	myoadenylate stain

connective tissue proliferation in muscle (see Figure 8-4). Additional histologic stains which are useful include the oil red O stain for lipids (see Figure 9-11) and the periodic acid Schiff stain for glycogen.

Fiber Types

Human muscle fibers differ with respect to histochemical staining, ultrastructural detail, biochemical and physiological properties. With the myofibrillar ATPase reaction (pH 9.4) two major types of muscle fibers are identified: lightly staining type I's and dark type II's (see Figure 2-6). These two fiber types differ principally in their biochemical machinery for handling energy substrates. Type I's are more suited to oxidize tricarboxylic-acid-cycle substrates, ketone bodies, and free fatty acids. On the other hand, type II fibers are better equip-

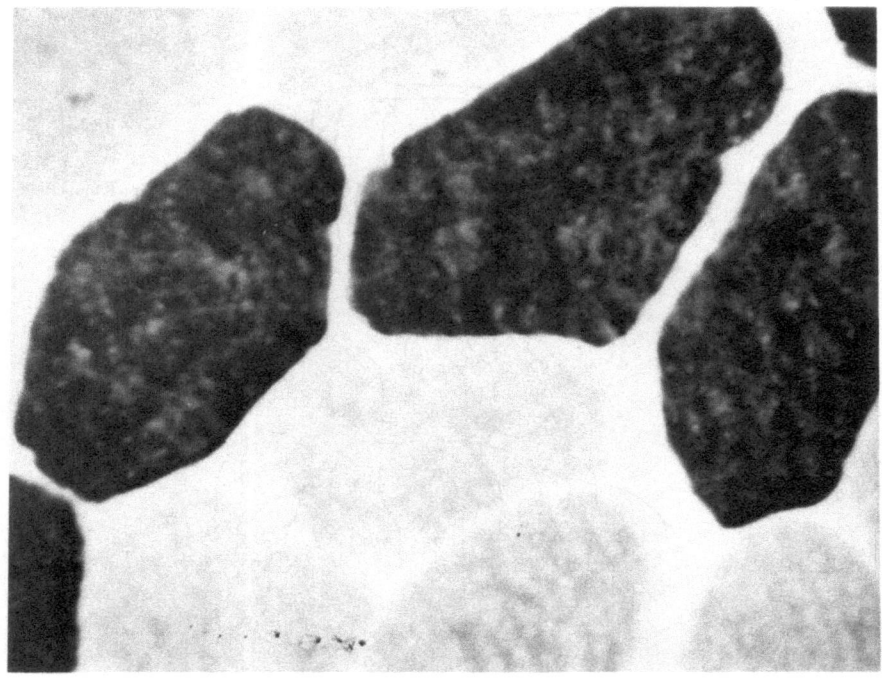

Figure 2-6.   The ATPase reaction.

ped for glycogenolysis and anaerobic glycolysis, and have more stored glycogen. These biochemical distinctions are directed by the innervating lower motor neuron. When a type I motor neuron inneravates a cluster of embryonic muscle fibers (myotubes) it influences their biochemical and physiologic properties (via "trophic factors") so that they all become type I muscle fibers. Type II motor neurons, by similar mechanisms, influence the development of myotubes to type II muscle fibers. As a result, fibers of the same motor unit are of a uniform histochemical type. If the neural supply of a motor unit is disrupted, the "orphaned" muscle fibers will either degenerate or will be reinnervated by nerve twigs from neighboring axons. If collateral sprouting occurs so that a type I nerve twig reinnervates a type II muscle fiber, the latter will be converted to a type I fiber (since it is now under the influence of type I "trophic factors"). Disruption of the nerve supply (deinnervation) with reinnervation leads to the phenomenon of type grouping (see Figure 2-7). Normally, muscle fascicles consist of a checkerboard pattern of the two fiber types. With type grouping, this

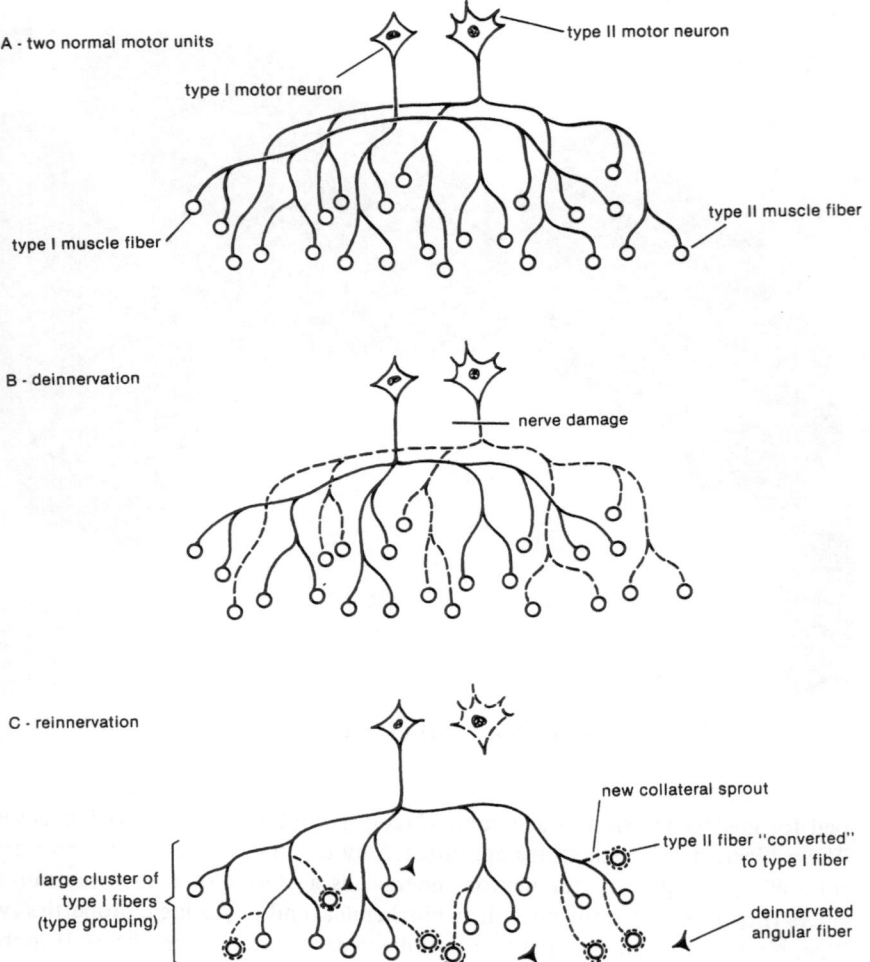

A - two normal motor units

type II motor neuron

type I motor neuron

type II muscle fiber

type I muscle fiber

B - deinnervation

nerve damage

C - reinnervation

new collateral sprout

type II fiber "converted" to type I fiber

large cluster of type I fibers (type grouping)

deinnervated angular fiber

Figure 2-7. Deinnervation and reinnervation.

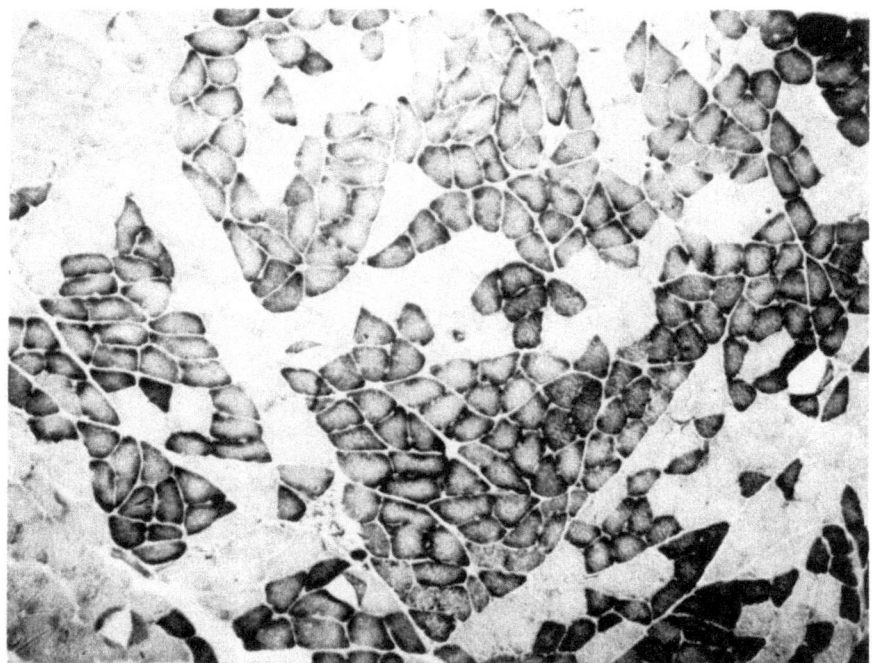

Figure 2-8. Type grouping (NADH-TR reaction). Muscle fascicles normally contain type I and II fibers in a mosaic pattern. With type grouping, this checkerboard appearance is replaced by clusters of single fiber types.

mosaic pattern is replaced by clusters of the same fiber type (see Figure 2-8). Type grouping implies chronic neuropathic disease; its electrical counterpart is the giant motor unit potential.

Histochemical Reaction

Histochemical methods in the study of muscle biopsies are the value for several reasons. They demonstrate specific fiber types on the basis of various enzyme reactions (i.e., ATPase); they may show an absence of a particular enzyme (i.e., phosphorylase), or they may reveal structural changes in the fibers (i.e., enzyme deficient cores with the NADH-TR reaction) (see Figure 5-4). Among the most useful of the histochemical stains are the myofibrillar adenosine triphosphates (ATPase), the NADH-tetrazolium reductase, the alkaline phosphatase and esterase reactions.

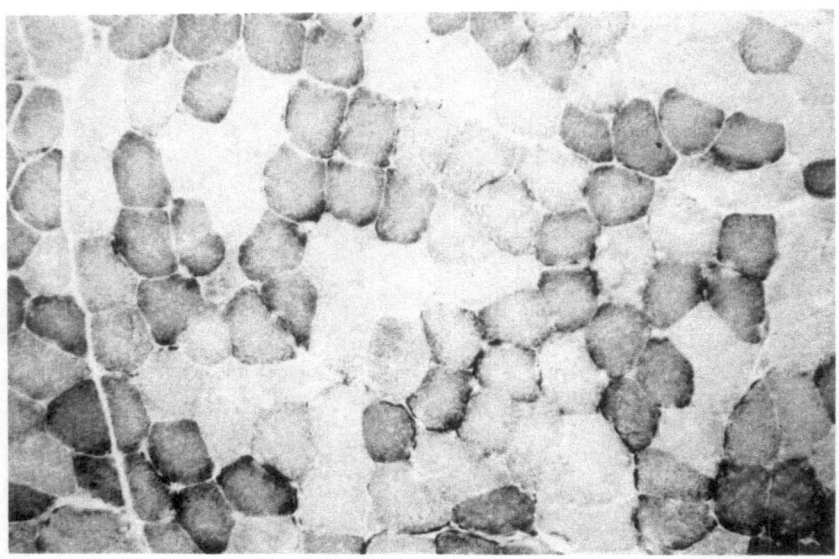

Figure 2-9. The NADH-TR reaction. A normal NADH-TR stain showing darkly stained type I fibers and lightly stained type II fibers. Because there are some intermediate staining fibers with this reaction, the ATPase stain is preferred for fiber typing.

The routine ATPase reaction (pH 9.4) is the standard stain for fiber typing. Because it sharply demarcates the two fiber types, (type I's appear light and II's dark) (see Figure 2-6), it is an excellent stain for demonstrating grouping. By adjusting the pH of the incubating media (reverse ATPase) one can change the staining characteristics of the fiber types. This is sometimes helpful in demonstrating grouping in fiber subtypes.

The NADH-tetrazolium reductase reaction stains type I fibers darkly and type II's lightly. The intermyofibrillar network comprising mitochondria and sarcoplasmic reticulum is well demonstrated (see Figure 2-9). The stain is of greatest value in looking for cores (see Figure 5-4), target fibers, tubular aggregates, and other cytoarchitectural changes.

Positive staining with the alkaline phosphatase reaction has been found to be characteristic of a particular fiber type. Normal fibers are unstained (pale yellow) while abnormal fibers are stained black. These fibers are probably undergoing early degeneration or are in a certain stage of regeneration ("regen-degen" fibers) (Engel and Cunningham, 1970) (see Figure 2-10). Such fibers are frequently seen in primary myopathies (polymyositis and the dystrophies).

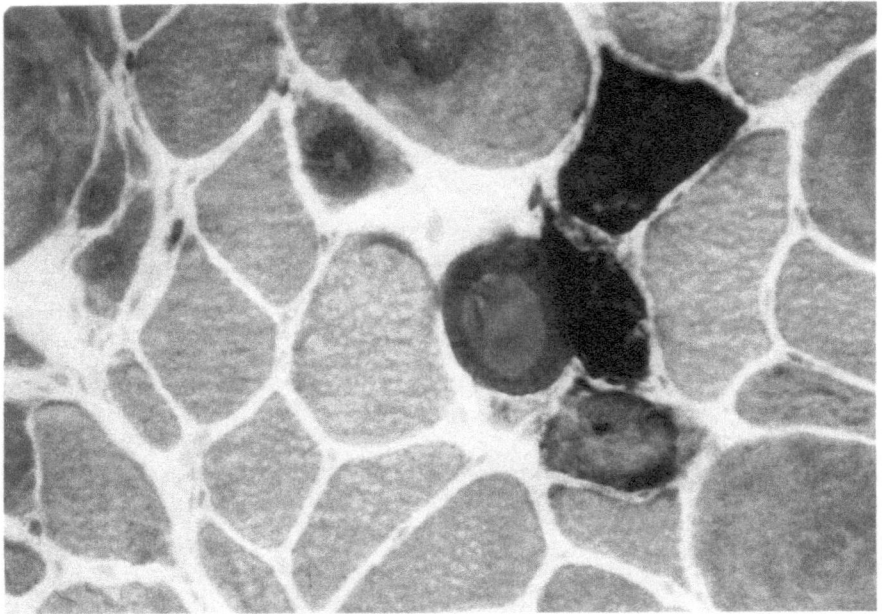

Figure 2-10. The alkaline phosphatase reaction. The paler staining fibers are normal and the darkly staining ones are "regen-degen" fibers.

In addition, positive staining (black) of the connective tissue with this reaction is evidence of the increased fibroblast activity that occurs in polymyositis (Engel, unpublished observation).

The esterase stain highlights deinnervated fibers which appear dark and angulated (see Figure 2-11). Macrophages and motor end plates are also darkly stained with the esterase reaction.

Myopathic Versus Neurogenic Changes

A summary of morphologic changes characteristic of myopathic and neuropathic processes is presented in Table 2-6.

Before leaving the topic of biopsy, just a brief word regarding nerve histology must be added. To date, nerve biopsy has not been as rewarding a procedure as muscle biopsy. Part of the problem is that only the sural nerve (a pure sensory nerve) is available for examination. Nerve biopsy is helpful when a suspected neuropathy has a distinctive histological picture (i.e., vasculitis, amyloidosis, sarcoidosis, leprosy, inflammatory polyradiculoneuropathy, metachro-

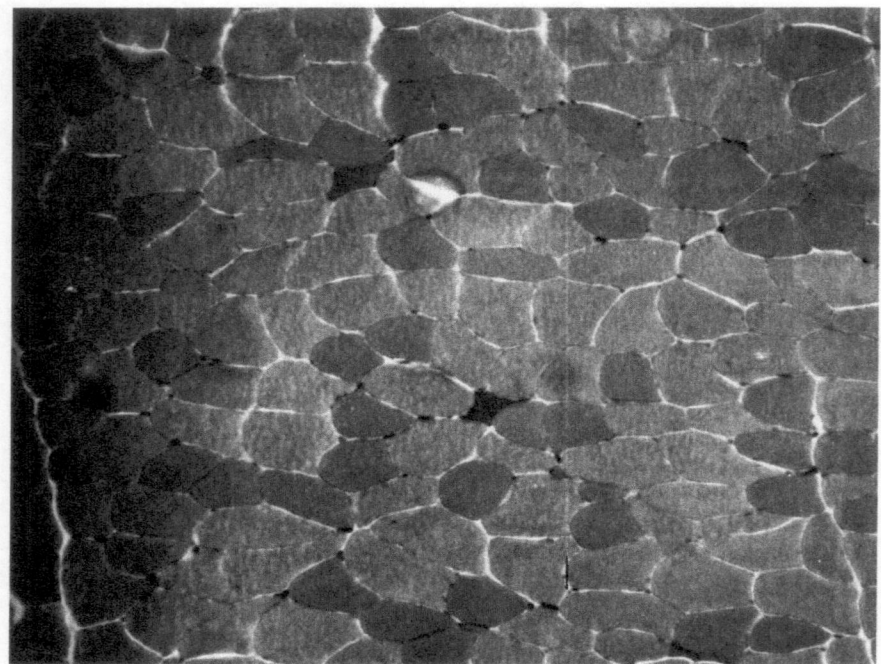

Figure 2-11. The esterase reaction. Darkly staining angular fibers are seen in this biopsy, indicating acute denervation.

matic leukodystrophy, and Krabbe's disease). Discussion of the specific morphologic abnormalities seen in these entities is beyond the scope of this book.

OTHER STUDIES

Creatine Phosphokinase

Determination of serum creatine phosphokinase (CPK) levels is a useful screening procedure when one suspects neuromuscular disease. The most striking elevations occur in the dystrophies (especially the Duchenne and Becker varieties), in myositis (from whatever cause), and in cases of malignant hyperthermia. An elevated CPK, however, does not necessarily imply primary muscle disease nor does a normal value necessarily exclude one. Mildly increased CPK concentrations are characteristic of the spinal muscular atrophies and amyo-

Table 2-8. CPK Isoenzymes in Various Tissues

	Percent MM	Percent MB	Percent BB
adult skeletal muscle	99	< 1	≪ 1
adult cardiac muscle	76	22	2
brain	< 1	< 1	99

trophic lateral sclerosis (neurogenic diseases). Physical exercise, if prolonged and severe, may also elevate the CPK, sometimes to astronomical levels. (Some of the highest CPK's recorded are found in epileptics after a series of seizures.) In some myopathies and junctional disorders, the CPK is normal. Typically, patients with periodic paralysis and disorders of muscle energy metabolism have normal values when they are asymptomatic.

Creatine phosphokinase levels are also of value in screening for carrier states in certain hereditary myopathies (see Chapter 4) and for monitoring disease activity in the inflammatory myopathies (see Chapter 8).

Creatine phosphokinase is the enzyme that transfers a high energy phosphate from creatine phosphate to ADP, forming creatine and ATP. It allows muscle to rapidly mobilize its storage pool of high energy phosphate bonds.

Creatine phosphokinase occurs as a dimmer. Since there are two subunits, there are three isoenzymes (MM, MB and BB). In the normal adult the serum CPK is over ninety percent MM isoenzyme with little MB and even less BB forms. These three isoenzymes originate from different tissues. The MM form is derived chiefly from skeletal muscle while CPK-MB is mostly of cardiac origin. The BB isoenzyme has its origin in brain, genitourinary and gastrointestinal tissues (see Table 2-8).

Relative amounts of the isoenzymes change with the maturation of muscle tissue. In fetal muscle only the BB form is found up to the sixth week of gestation. By week 12, there is no longer any CPK-BB and the MB variety is the major isoenzyme. CPK-MM appears by week 8 and after week 12 is the predominant isoenzyme. Vigorous fusion of the myoblasts to form myotubes appears to be associated with the rapid production of the MM form. At birth, human skeletal muscle has essentially the adult type distribution of isoenzymes with little or no BB, some MB and mostly MM.

In neuromuscular diseases, elevated CPK levels reflect pathologic leakage of mature muscle fibers. In some myopathies, the increased serum CPK concentration contains a disproprotionately high percentage of CPK-BB. This probably reflects leakage from immature or regenerating muscle fibers and is seen in patients whose biopsies show abundant "regen-degen" fibers with the alkaline phosphatase stain (Zweig et al, 1980).

Other "muscle enzymes" including aldolase, aminotransferases (GOT,

GPT), and lactate dehydrogenase may be elevated in neuromuscular diseases. However, serum determination of these enzymes seems to add little to the information already provided by the CPK concentration.

Ischemic Exercise Test/Fasting

For information on ischemic exercise test/fasting, the reader is directed to Chapter 9.

SUMMARY

Electromyographic studies and muscle biopsy are the key procedures for identifying the specific cause of a neuromuscular complaint. Once the diagnosis has been clearly established, the physician can concentrate his efforts on appropriate therapy. The nine chapters that follow discuss specific muscle disorders with special emphasis on their management and treatment.

CHAPTER 3

Disorders of Neuromuscular Transmission

ANATOMY AND PHYSIOLOGY OF THE NEUROMUSCULAR JUNCTION

To understand better the disorders of the neuromuscular junction (NMJ) some basic knowledge of the anatomy and physiology of this region must first be mastered. The neuromuscular junction (Figure 3-1) consists of a motor nerve ending (presynaptic terminal) and a postsynaptic muscle fiber membrane separated by a space, the synaptic cleft. The motor nerve terminal is filled with packets called synaptic vesicles, which contain acetycholine (ACh), the chemical transmitter. Each vesicle contains a quantum of ACh, which is estimated to be between 10^3 and 10^4 ACh molecules (Hartzell et al. 1976). At rest, the muscle membrane is charged, being relatively more negative on the inside compared to the outside. This resting membrane potential, which measures approximately -80 mV, arises because:

1. the membrane at rest is more permeable to K^+ than to Na^+;
2. an active transport mechanism maintains the internal Na^+ concentration at a low level;
3. the membrane is impermeable to organic anions within the cell.

Normally, small amounts of transmitter (ACh) are spontaneously released vai exocytosis into the synaptic cleft. After diffusing across the cleft, the ACh combines with glycoprotein receptors located on the surface of the post-synaptic membrane. These receptors are believed to control the gateway of ion specific membrane pores. The interaction between ACh and its receptor changes the permeability of the postsynaptic membrane to Na^+ and K^+ (Takeuchi and Takeuchi, 1960) so that the permeability to both ions is increased but much more so for the former than the latter ion. As a result Na^+ moves into the cell and the resting membrane potential becomes slightly more positive (by 0.75 to

41

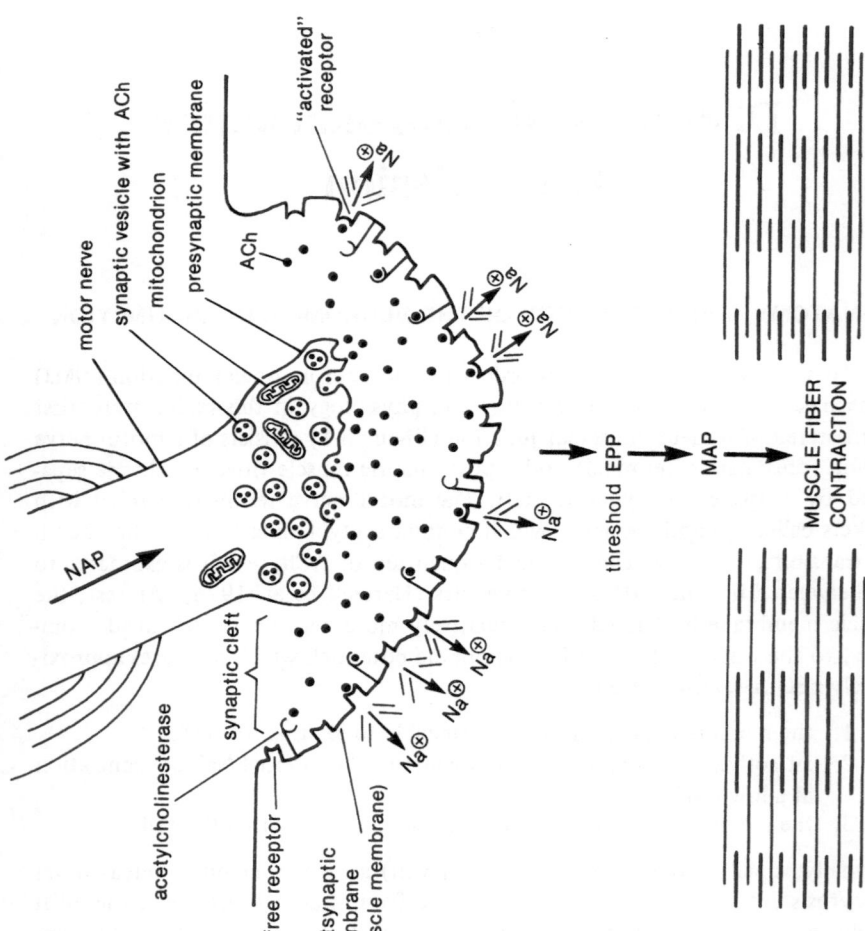

Figure 3-1. The neuromuscular junction and neuromuscular transmission.

1.35 mV). These spontaneous small changes in potential recorded at the post-synaptic membrane are called miniature end plate potentials (MEPPs). They are purely a local phenomenon and are not propagated along the muscle fiber membrane. On the other hand, when the motor nerve is stimulated by a nerve action potential (NAP), numerous quanta of ACh are liberated. Via similar permeability changes described above, a much greater change in potential is produced, called an end plate potential (EPP). The EPP, if above threshold (i.e., of sufficient magnitude to change the membrane potential from -80 mV to -55 mV), triggers the generation of a muscle action potential (MAP) (Figure 3-1). The muscle action potential is propagated along the muscle fiber without decay of its amplitude, and is transmitted to the interior of the fiber by means of an elaborate system of membrane infoldings called the transverse tubules. Once propagated to the interior, it triggers muscle fiber contraction (see Chapter 2 for details).

It is of importance that the amplitude of the end plate potential depends on the number of ACh molecules that interact with postsynaptic receptors. Generally only a small portion of such molecules released in response to a nerve action potential interacts with receptors and only a small fraction of receptors is "activated" at any one time (Katz and Miledi, 1973). The number of successful interactions between ACh and receptor is thus a matter of probability, and under normal conditions, the number of such interactions is more than adequate to trigger a muscle action potential. This excess is referred to as the safety margin of neuromuscular transmission (Drachman, 1978). Many agents, such as curare, combine with the same receptors as ACh. By doing so, they decrease the number of available receptors and, therefore may diminish the end plate potential to subthreshold values.

The number of quanta released in response to a nerve stimulus (NAP) and thus the magnitude of the end plate potential can also be influenced by the chemical environment of the junction. If one decreases the concentration of Ca^{++} or increases that of Mg^{++} in this region, the number of quanta released for a given stimulus is reduced.

The entire process of neuromuscular transmission is rapid, requiring only milliseconds. Depolarization of the postsynaptic membrane is terminated by the removal of ACh from the cleft. This is accomplished principally by the action of an enzyme, acetylcholinesterase, located at the postsynaptic region. This enzyme hydrolyzes ACh to choline and acetic acid, neither of which is active as a chemical transmitter.

Disorders of neuromuscular transmission, therefore, may result from either pre- or postsynaptic abnormalities. Presynaptic disorders are those in which an insufficient number of ACh packets are released in response to a nerve action potential. This is the underlying pathophysiology in the Eaton-Lambert syndrome, botulism, and possibly tick paralysis. Postsynaptic blockade of neuromuscular transmission occurs when ACh is not permitted to combine with its receptor. This will occur if the receptor is destroyed or if some other substance is occupying its active site. Such situations occur in myasthenia gravis and curare poisoning. Furthermore, failure of acetylcholinesterase to terminate the action of ACh may also impair transmission.

The sections which follow briefly discuss some of the more common disorders of neuromuscular transmission, including the Eaton-Lambert syndrome, botulism, tick paralysis, and myasthenia gravis.

THE EATON-LAMBERT SYNDROME (MYASTHENIC SYNDROME)

In 1961, Lambert and co-workers first described a characteristic neuromuscular transmission defect in patients with bronchiogenic carcinoma. It is now recognized that this disorder, called the Eaton-Lambert syndrome, may occur in association with a variety of malignancies including those of the breast, prostate, stomach, and rectum (Brain and Henson, 1958). Small cell bronchogenic carcinoma accounts for approximately 50 to 60 percent of the total cases. Overall, 70 percent of patients with the Eaton-Lambert syndrome will harbor a malignancy (Elmqvist and Lambert, 1968). Neuromuscular symptoms commonly precede those of the underlying carcinoma sometimes by as long as three years. Exceptionally, symptoms appear after the successful removal and treatment of the neoplasm. There seems to be no relation between the course of the neuromuscular syndrome and that of the tumor.

Becasue of the frequent association of neoplasia and the Eaton-Lambert syndrome, it has been proposed that the defect in neuromuscular transmission is produced by a circulating "carcinotoxin" synthesized by the tumor. Ishikawa et al (1977) produced the identical neuromuscular transmission defect in vitro by exposing frog nerve-muscle preps to tumor extracts derived from a patient with bronchiogenic carcinoma and the Eaton-Lambert syndrome.

In 30 percent of patients with the Eaton-Lambert syndrome, a neoplasm is never found even after long-term follow-up. Some of these patients have subsequently developed autoimmune disorders including hyperthyroidism (Norris 1966), hypothryroidism (Gutmann, 1972) and Sjögren's syndrome (Brown et al, 1968). This association and the recent observations that such patients may improve with immunosuppressive therapies imply that an altered immune state may be the underlying problem.

Clinical Presentation: Signs and Symptoms

The Eaton-Lambert syndrome occurs most commonly in males over 40 years of age. The principal symptoms are weakness and easy fatigability of the proximal muscles of the lower extremities and hip girdle. [This weakness differs from that of myasthenia gravis in being worse soon after arising, and improving as the day wears on.] Early complaints include difficulty in rising from a chair and in climbing stairs. Mild aching of the thighs, dryness of the mouth, and distal paresthesias are frequently found at this stage. In contrast ot myasthenia gravis, symptoms of involvement of the ocular, bulbar, and neck musculature either do not occur or are mild and transient, and are seldom present at the time of the initial evaluation. Ptosis, diplopia, dysphagia, and dysarthria, so prominent in myasthenia gravis, are rarely bothersome in the Eaton-Lambert syndrome. In addition, impaired cholinergic autonomic function including dry mouth, impaired lacrimation and sweating, non-reactive pupils, and impotence may occur in the Eaton-Lambert syndrome. However, dysautonomia is rarely encountered in myasthenia gravis.

Careful manual testing of muscles often reveals a delay in the development of strength at the onset of maximal muscle contraction. Strength seems to improve with repetitive efforts; however, with prolonged sustained activity of the muscle, the weakness reappears. Tendon reflexes are usually diminished or absent. Other neurologic syndromes associated with carcinoma (Teravainen and Larsen, 1977) including peripheral neuropathy, cerebellar ataxia, and myositis may be found in these patients.

Laboratory Studies

Serum muscle enzymes

Serum muscle enzymes are normal in the Eaton-Lambert syndrome unless there is an accompanying myositis (see Chapter 8).

Electrodiagnostic tests

In the Eaton-Lambert syndrome, there is a characteristic response of muscle to repetitive nerve stimulation which is the key to identification of the disorder and to its differentiation from myasthenia gravis. Typically, patients with the syndrome have (McQuillen and Johns, 1967):

1. an abnormally low amplitude of the compound motor action potential to a single stimulus,

2. a decremental response at low rates (1-3/sec) of nerve stimulation, and

3. marked facilitation of the response at high rates of stimulation (20-50/ sec) and after 10 seconds the maximal muscle contraction (see Figure 3-2).

The characteristic EMG changes can be identified at an accessible peripheral site (i.e., abducton minimi digiti muscle) in all cases, although on clinical grounds, features are evident only in proximal muscles. It is important to note that in most centers, neuromuscular transmission studies are not done as part of

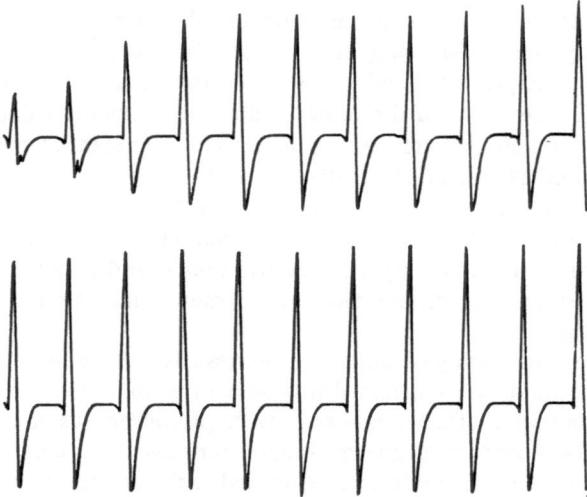

Figure 3-2. Characteristic EMG in the Eaton-Lambert syndrome. Note the increasing amplitude of the muscle action potentials at high frequency stimulation (20/sec).

the routine EMG study. Thus, unless the electromyographer is informed that the Eaton-Lambert syndrome is a diagnostic consideration, the characteristic electrical findings may be missed.

Muscle biopsy

Microscopic examination of muscle tissue is not helpful in diagnosing the myasthenic syndrome. Biopsies of such patients may reveal type II fiber atrophy which is probably secondary to the functional block of neuromuscular transmission and disuse. Electron microscopic studies of the neuromuscular junction typically show overdevelopment of the postsynaptic folds which is in direct contrast to the changes in myasthenia gravis.

Other

Unlike myasthenia gravis where the bedside administration of edrophonium (Tensilon) produces a marked but a transient increase in muscle strength, the Eaton-Lambert syndrome has a variable response to this drug. A positive or negative response to edrophonium neither supports nor refutes the diagnosis of the Eaton-Lambert syndrome.

Pathophysiology

In many respects, the defect in neuromuscular transmission in the myasthenic syndrome is like that produced by magnesium ions, botulinum toxin, and neomycin, agents whose predominant effect is to decrease the number of quanta of acetycholine (ACh) released by a nerve impulse. Intracellular recordings of affected muscles show that the amplitude of the miniature end plate potentials (MEPPs) are normal, but they are reduced in frequency. End plate potentials (EPPs) produced by an evoked response are reduced in amplitude. Because the ACh content and level of choline acetyltransferase activity are normal (Molenaar et al, 1982), the defect lies not in the synthesis or storage of transmitter, but in the mechanism of release itself (see Figure 3-3). Whether this reduction in transmitter release is the result of a circulating "carcinotoxin" or is mediated by an altered immune response remains to be determined. Recent observations that patients with Eaton-Lambert syndrome improve when treated with plasmapheresis and immunosuppressants (Dau and Denys, 1982) suggest that circulating factors such as auto antibodies may participate in its pathogenesis.

Course and Treatment

The prognosis in the myasthenic syndrome is largely determined by the associated carcinoma. Removal and treatment of the tumor has little or no effect on the accompanying neuromuscular disorder; thus treatment must be directed specifically to the transmission defect. Currently, guanidine hydrochloride is the most effective agent. It enhances ACh release and produces clinical and electrophysiologic improvement in the majority of patients with the disorder. The drug is not without side effects that include bone marrow depression and interstitial nephritis among others. Because of these side effects, it is recommended that the drug be started at low levels and gradually increased at weekly intervals to a maximum dose of 30-35 mg/kg/day. Monthly blood counts and periodic evaluation of renal function should also be done routinely. Other agents that also promote ACh release such as aminophylline, caffeine, and epinephrine have been found to produce improvement in a limited number of cases (Takamori et al, 1973). Steroids may be of benefit because they enhance NMJ transmission by stimulating ACh synthesis and release (Hall, 1983). Anticholinesterase drugs have a role in the treatment of the Eaton-Lambert syndrome. The role of plasmapheresis and immunosuppressive therapy awaits further clarification.

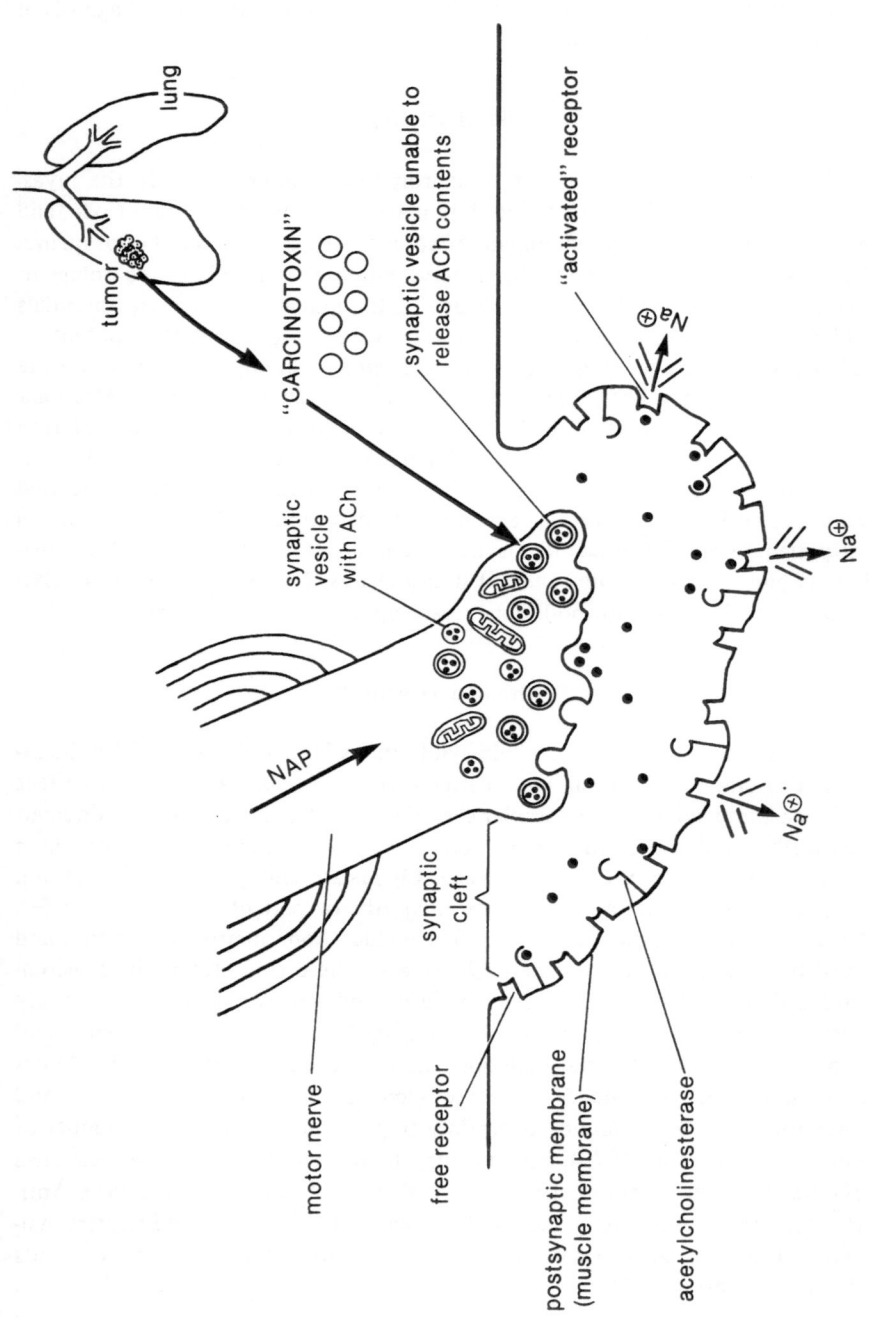

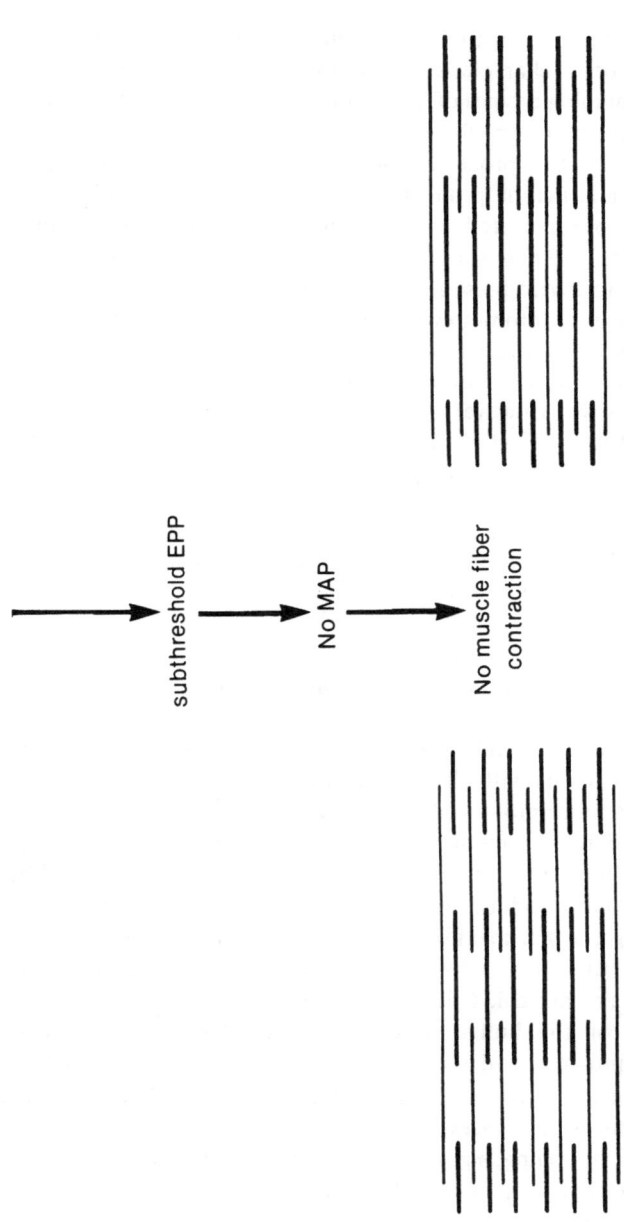

Figure 3-3. Diagrammatic representation of the pathophysiology of the Eaton-Lambert syndrome.

BOTULISM

Ingestion of or exposure to significant amounts of the exotoxin of Clostridium botulinum produces a characteristic symptom complex called botulism. While there are six immunologic types of Clostridium botulinum, botulism in man usually results from the toxins produced by types A, B and E. Type A and B toxin are found in inadequately processed meats, fruits, and vegetables. Type E is associated with fish and marine products. Additional cases of botulism, particularly type A, have bee reported as a complication of infected extremity wounds (Miller and Moses, 1977). The illness varies in severity from mild cases requiring no treatment to severe poisonings with profound weakness and respiratory failure. The clinical syndromes evoked by the different toxins, A, B and E, vary somewhat in their manifestations. All three interfere with acetycholine (ACh) release and thus impair transmission at neuromuscular junctions and autonomic cholinergic sites. However, in type A intoxication, the neuromuscular synapses are selectively affected and profound muscle weakness dominates the clinical picture. Ingestion of type B or E toxin, on the other hand, produces marked autonomic disturbances with little musculoskeletal impairment (Jenzer et al, 1975). Because each hour may be critical to the survival of the patient with botulism and for the prevention of other cases, prompt clinical, epidemiologic, and laboratory efforts are necessary.

Clinical Presentation: Signs and Symptoms

Onset of symptoms of botulism begins between six hours to eight days after the ingestion of toxin. Patients with short incubation periods are usually more severely affected, have a more prolonged course and a poorer prognosis. (Donadio et al, 1971). Type E toxin ingestion produces early and severe gastrointestinal manifestations with prominent nausea, vomiting, abdominal distention, and diarrhea. Type B toxin produces less of the above symptoms and type A even less. After this stage, ocular manifestations including blurred vision, diplopia, and ptosis appear. The pupils may be dilated and non-reactive; however, more commonly, they are normal. (Cherington, 1974). Ocular symptoms are followed by weakness of the bulbar muscles with resultant dysarthria and dysphagia. A rapidly progressive descending quadraparesis may immediately succeed the bulbar stage. Significant respiratory impairment will develop in approximately 30 percent of these cases.

With types B and E poisoning, signs and symptoms of autonomic dysfunction are promenent. Obstipation, urinary hesitancy, impairment of potency, orthostatic hypotension, and dry eyes and mouth are commonly seen.

Mental functions, somatic sensations, and tendon reflexes remain normal in all types of intoxication.

The diagnosis is not difficult when several members of a common household are affected, or if samples of the contaminated food are available for testing. Isolated cases of the disease, however, may be confused with poliomyelitis, myasthenia gravis, brainstem strokes, Guillain-Barré syndrome, Eaton-Lambert syndrome, or diphtheric polyneuritis (see Figure 1-1). A normal cerebrospinal fluid examination excludes poliomyelitis while the absence of sensory abnormalities, the prominent cranial nerve involvement, and the normal tendon reflexes speak against the Guillain-Barré syndrome. Myasthenia gravis is ruled out by the absence of fluctuations in strength and by electromyographic studies. The prominent ocular signs exclude the Eaton-Lambert syndrome and the lack of associated neurologic signs makes the diagnosis of branstem strokes unlikely. Appropriate electrical (EMG) and infectious disease studies eliminate Corynebacterium diphthriae as the causative agent.

The diagnosis is confirmed by injecting the patient's serum into normal mice and mice pretreated with antibotulinus serum. If the patient has botulism, the pretreated group of animals will survive while the former group will die within 48 hours of receiving the patient's serum.

Laboratory Studies

Serum muscle enzymes and muscle biopsy

Determination of serum levels of muscle enzymes is of no value in the diagnosis or management of botulism. Muscle biopsy shows changes compatible with structurally deinnervated muscle. This is presumably the result of physiologic deinnervation of the fibers secondary to disrupted neuromuscular transmission.

Electrodiagnostic tests

Electromyography is essential for confirming the diagnosis of a suspected case of botulism. However, one must keep in mind that EMG studies may be completely normal in the early stages of the disease despite obvious weakness (Cherington and Ryan, 1970; Hagenan and Muller-Jensen, 1978). Furthermore, cases of type B or E intoxication may never develop EMG changes (Jenzer et al, 1975).

The characteristic EMG abnormalities of botulism resemble those of the myasthenic syndrome and include (Gutmann and Pratt, 1976):

1. decreased amplitude of the compound motor action potential (CMAP) evoked by a single supramaximal nerve stimulus,

2. facilitation of the amplitude of the CMAP with rapid repetitive stimulation (>20/sec).

Botulism, however, differs from the Eaton-Lambert syndrome in several respects. At slow rates of repetitive stimulation (<3/sec), the amplitude of the evoked motor response characteristically decreases in the myasthenic syndrome. This is not always true in botulism. In addition, the facilitation response at high frequency stimulation is far more dramatic in the Eaton-Lambert syndrome than in botulism.

Pathophysiology

Botulism toxin inhibits the release of ACh at cholinergic transmission sites. The toxin probably interferes with a calcium binding mechanism necessary for transmitter release (Schiller and Stalberg, 1978). Why type B and E toxins preferentially affect autonomic cholinergic junctions while type A toxin selectively impairs transmission at neuromuscular synapses is not known.

Treatment and Prognosis

There are three major goals of therapy in botulism. These are:

1. removal of unabsorbed toxin from the gastrointestinal tract,
2. neutralization of circulating toxin by administering antitoxin,
3. compensation of the neuromuscular blockade by the use of mechanical ventilators and pharmacologic agents.

The most immediate danger to the patient with botulism is respiratory failure. Monitoring the patient's respiratory status with serial determination of the arterial blood gases, vital capacity, and pulmonary functions, is necessary. Patients with evidence of bulbar involvement should be hospitalized and placed in an intensive care setting. Mechanical respirators are used if significant respiratory impairment develops.

If the food suspected of causing the illness was recently ingested, an emetic should be administered.

Because all antitoxins are of equine origin and there is a possibility of anaphylaxis, such therapy should be reserved for severe cases. Testing for sensitivity to the antitoxin should always precede its use. Trivalent ABE antitoxin is given in cases where the specific type is unknown.

Guanidine hydrocholoride in doses of 15-35 mg/kg/day (Cherington and Ryan, 1970) may produce marked clinical improvement in some patients. The use of this drug may allow the patient to get by without a respirator, thus avoiding the additional complications which attend such therapy.

The prognosis for survival is good even in severe poisoning if adequate supportive care is provided. Recovery in survivors may be prolonged but is nearly complete in all instances. Patients with milder degrees of poisoning are usually back to normal in two to three months, while more severe intoxications may require a year or more for full recovery. The appropriate public health officials should be notified in all cases.

TICK PARALYSIS

A peculiar type of ascending motor paralysis has been observed in animals and humans bitten by the Rocky Mountain wood tick, Dermacentor andersoni. Only the female insect, which produces a neurotoxin in its salivary glands, is capable of producing tick paralysis. While the illness is uncommon and confined to the northwestern sectors of North America, recognition of this entity in a stricken patient can be lifesaving.

Clinical Presentation: Signs and Symptoms

Tick paralysis usually begins five to six days after the insect has embedded itself in the skin. The hairline seems to be a particularly favored site of feeding. Weakness appears initially in the lower extremities and rapidly increases to involve the upper limbs and bulbar musculature. Respiratory impairment is the primary cause of death in fatal cases. Examination of patients with tick paralysis most frequently reveals a flaccid quadriparesis, absent tendon reflexes, and sensory abnormalities in the distal extremities. Differential diagnosis includes Guillain-Barré syndrome, periodic paralysis, and spinal cord compression (spinal shock) (see Figure 1-1).

Laboratory Studies and Pathophysiology

Electromyography

Electrophysiologic studies on patients with tick paralysis suggest that the toxin inhibits the release of acetycholine from the presynaptic motor nerve terminals (Murnaghan 1960). This toxin seems to act specifically on the neuromuscular junction and does not effect autonomic cholinergic synapses. In addition, the toxin may also impair conduction in peripheral nerves (Cherington and Snyder, 1968).

Treatment

Removal of the tick before a moribund state develops results in a rapid and full recovery of function (Emmons and McLennan, 1959). This should be done with extreme care to insure that the entire insect including the embedded head is removed. Applying a lighted match to the tick prior to removing it with forceps seems to be the most preferred method.

MYASTHENIA GRAVIS

Myasthenia gravis (MG) is a disorder of neuromuscular transmission manifested by weakness and fatigability of voluntary muscles. In recent years, it has become evident that this disorder is one of the foremost examples of autoimmune disease in man.

Myasthenia gravis is not an uncommon disease. In a populace the size of the greater Washington, D.C. area (approximately three million) one can expect to find over 120 cases of the disease with twelve new cases appearing annually. The illness may affect people of any age or of either sex. However, there appears to be two ages of peak incidence: for women, the third decade, and for men, the fifth and sixth decades. Overall, women are affected twice as frequently as men but the female:male ratio changes from 4.5:1 in myasthenia beginning before the age of 30 to an equal incidence when the disease begins in later life (Simpson, 1978).

Myasthenia may vary in severity from a mild nonprogressive disorder limited to the extraocular muscles to a rapidly progressive and fatal illness. With proper management, the patient with MG can have a meaningful existence with few limitations.

Clinical Presentation: Signs and Symptoms

The most important clinical feature of MG is muscle weakness worsened by exercise and relieved by rest. In about 50 percent of cases, the disease begins in the extraocular muscles with resultant diplopia and ptosis. Approximately 30 percent of patients have bulbar symptoms (dysarthria and dysphagia) as the initial manifestation, while the remaining cases start with proximal limb weakness. In most instances, the disease ultimately involves the cranial nerve musculature as well as the muscles of the proximal extremities and neck. Chewing, swallowing, holding up the head, climbing stairs, and rising from a chair are particularly troublesome tasks. Ptosis is common and may vary from one eye to another (a feature which is probably pathognomonic for myasthenia gravis). Subtle ptosis can be brought out or accentuated by having the patient sustain upgaze. Extraocular muscle involvement does not follow any particular pattern. Paresis of a single eye muscle or total external ophthalmoplegia may occur. The motility pattern may mimic an internuclear ophthalmoplegia (INO) with failure of the adducting eye to move beyond the midline and with dissociated nystagmus in the abducting eye on attempted lateral gaze. This pseudo-INO is distinguished from a true INO (signifying disease of the medial longitudinal fasciculus) by the fact that in the former, the adducting paresis and nystagmus develop only after sustained horizonal gaze. Both features increase in severity as the eccentric eye position is held. With a true INO, the adducting paresis and nystagmus appear as soon as the eyes reach the eccentric gaze position, and is unchanging in amplitude. Furthermore, edrophonium may "cure" the pseudo-INO but has no effect on the true INO.

Respiratory muscles are frequently affected and respiratory failure poses a real threat to many myasthenics. In addition, as many as 40 percent of patients have electrocardiographic and/or kinetocardiographic evidence of myocardial involvement (Patten, 1978).

While most patients who present with ocular manifestations go on to develop generalized MG, a small group will have the disease forever restricted to the ocular muscles. This ocular form of MG comprises approximately 16 percent (Grob et al, 1981) of patients with MG. There is not complete agreement whether ocular MG is actually a limited form of MG or a separate illness. The facts that the ocular variety occurs more commonly in males, has an older mean age of onset (38 years as compared to 28 years in generalized MG), and has a higher spontaneous remission rate (30 percent as compared to 11 percent in generalized MG), support the separatists' view. The restricted ocular form can present diagnostic problems and may be confused with dysthyroid myopathy. The differentiation between the two is aided, however, by the fact that ptosis is common in ocular MG but is only rarely encountered in thyroid eye disease. Also, weakness of the orbicularis oculi is not a feature of dysthyroid myopathy, but is very common in ocular MG.

In MG there are few physical signs aside from the weakness and fatigability of the involved muscles. The tendon relexes are normal or hyperactive, but if the reflex is repeatedly elicited, the response may progressively decline until it disappears. Persistent absence of knee and ankle jerks suggests that the weakness is caused by carcinomatous myasthenia rather than by MG (see Table 3-1). Signs of neuronal dysfunction such as sensory changes and fasciculations are not found. Ten to fifteen percent of babies born to myasthenic mothers have an evanescent form of the illness. This neonatal variety presents at birth and persists for up to 12 weeks. The baby is hypotonic and has difficulty breathing, swallowing, and suckling (see Figure 5-1). This neonatal form provided an early clue to the pathophysiology of the disorder. Several (non-autoimmune) varieties of the diseas that differ from classical MG in their clinical characteristics and pathophysiology have been described (see Table 3-2). It is important to recognize this unique subgroup of myasthenics because thymectomy is certainly of no value to these patients.

Pathophysiology

The observed similarity between MG and curare poisoning pointed first to the neuromuscular junction as the region of abnormality. Electrophysiologic studies on myasthenics supported the concept of impaired synaptic transmission as

Table 3-1. Comparison of the Eaton-Lambert Syndrome with Myasthenia Gravis

	Eaton-Lambert Syndrome	Myasthenia Gravis
clinical features		
age of onset	40 years or later	any age
sex distribution (♂/♀)	5:1	3:5
symptoms of weakness	difficulty in walking, rising from chair, stepping, and climbing down	fluctuating ptosis, diplopia, dysphagia, difficulty chewing, thick speech
distribution of weakness	proximal limbs (LE > UE)	ocular muscles, lids, oropharyn neck flexors, proximal limbs
muscle pain and tenderness	present	absent
tendon reflexes	diminished or absent	normal or increased
resting muscle strength	reduced	normal or near normal
effect or repeated activity	strength increases, then decreases	decrease in strength
associated diseases	pulmonary carcinoma and other malignancies	thymomas and autoimmune disorders
EMG characteristics		
Single stimulus, rested muscle	CMAP and contraction reduced	CMAP and contraction normal
slow repetitive stimulation (1-3/sec)	CMAP and contraction decrease	CMAP and contraction decline
rapid repetitive stimulation (10-50/sec)	CMAP and contraction increase	CMAP and contraction decline
pathophysiology	Presynaptic: decrease in number of ACh packets released	Postsynaptic: ACh receptor blockade
treatment		
anticholinesterases	Mild or no improvement	improvement
guanidine	improvement	mile or no improvement

Table 3-2. Nonautoimmune Varieties of Myasthenia Gravis

	Clinical Features	Laboratory	Pathophysiology
classic autoimmune MG	sporadic fluctuating weakness of ocular, bulbar, and proximal limb muscles responsive to ancholinesterases and steroids	abnormal RNS elevated AChR-ab titers	antibody blockade of AChR and accelerated degradation of AChR
Acetylcholinesterase deficiency/reduced ACh release syndrome (Engel et al, 1977)	autosomal recessive fluctuating weakness of bulbar and proximal limb muscles but with decreased tendon reflexes unresponsive to anticholinesterases	abnormal RNS normal AChR-ab titers	diminished acetyl cholinesterase and reduced ACh release
slow channel syndrome (Engel et al, 1982)	autosomal dominant weakness of ocular, cervical, proximal and distal upper extremities unresponsive to anticholinesterases and steroids	abnormal RNS abnormal muscle biopsy normal AChR-ab titers	prolonged open time of ACh-induction channel

RNS = repetitive nerve stimulation.
ACh = acetylcholine.
AChR = acetylcholine receptor.
AChR-ab = acetylcholine receptor antibody.

the underlying cause of the disorder. Initially it was believed that the transmission failure resulted from inadequate ACh release in response to nerve action potentials. However, several observations correctly localized the abnormality to the postsynaptic region.

First it was demonstrated that the postsynaptic membranes of myasthenics, as compared with those of normal people, exhibit diminished binding of α-bungarotoxin (a component of snake venom with specific binding affinity for acetylcholine receptors) (Fambrough et al, 1973). Then an experimental animal model with the number of available acetylcholine receptor (ACh-R) sites reduced by pharmacologic blockade, was produced and it mimicked all the typical features of human MG (Satyamurti et al, 1975). Finally, direct electron microscopic visualization of the neuromuscular junctions of myasthenics confirmed that the presynaptic terminals were normal but that the postsynaptic areas exhibited marked morphologic abnormalities (Woolf, 1966; Engle and Santa, 1971). Thus it became evident that the abnormality in MG resided at the postsynaptic membrane and was due to a reduced number of available ACh-R sites.

An autoimmune was suspected because of several factors:

1. the increased association of autoimmune diseases in myasthenics,

2. the high incidence of thymic abnormalities in such patients [ten to 15 percent harbor thymomas while almost 60 percent have hyperplasia of the germinal centers] . (Castleman, 1966) (see Figure 3-4),

3. the presence of acetylcholine receptor antibody in a high percentage of patients with the disease.

Currently it is postulated that the disease results from an autoimmune response initiated in the thymus gland. The thymus contains in addition to lymphocytes, muscle-like myoid cells (epithelial cells). These cells have ACh-R protein similar to that found in skeletal muscle. Some alteration in thymic lymphocytes, possibly incited by a thymic tumor or vital infection, causes ACh-R specific T helper cells to become sensitized to ACh-R antigen of the myoid cell. This ultimately results in the production of circulating acetycholine receptor antibodies which block receptor sites and accelerate receptor degradation (Drachman et al, 1978). This same immunoglobulin is probably responsible for the passive transfer of the disease from man to mice and from myasthenic mothers to their neonates (Figure 3-5).

Thus the weakness in MG results from failure of neuromuscular transmission at many junctions because of the reduction of available ACh receptors. Receptor blockade diminishes the probability of successful interaction with ACh. Consequently, end plate potentials in some fibers are subthreshold and fail to trigger muscle action potentials and muscle fiber contraction. The power of the whole muscle is thereby reduced.

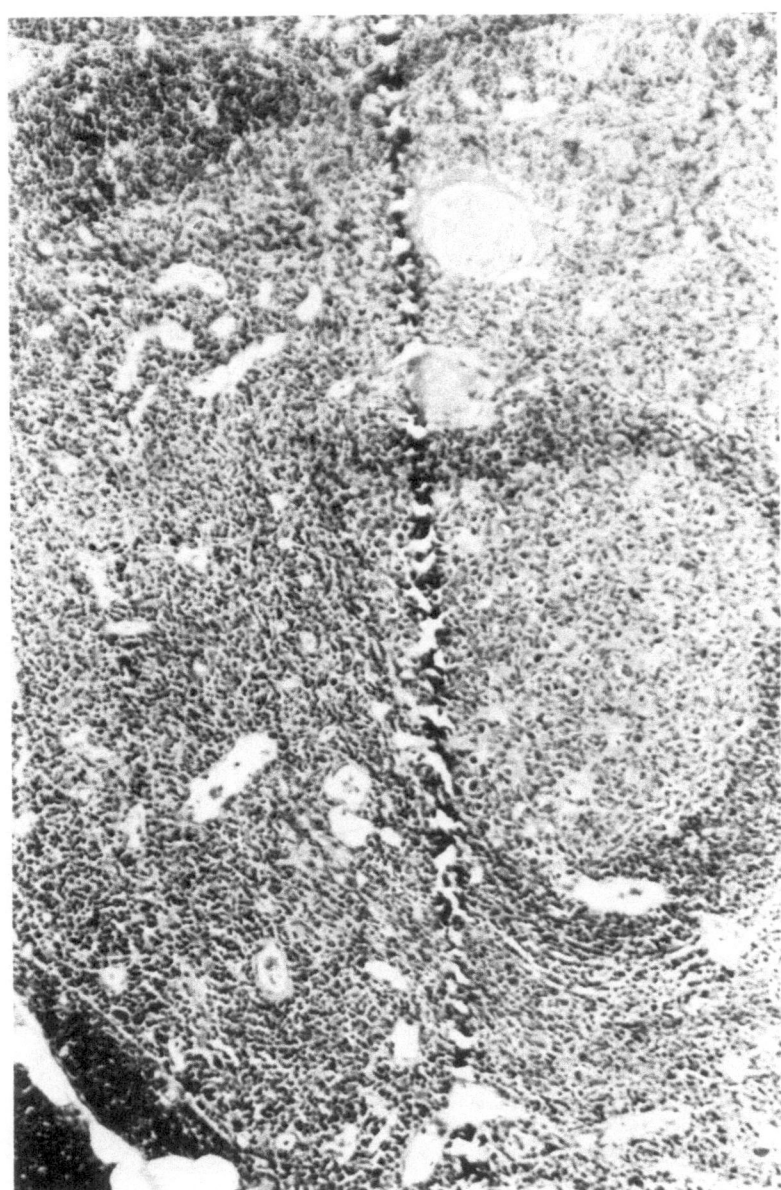

Figure 3-4. Hyperplastic thymus gland in patient with myasthenia gravis.

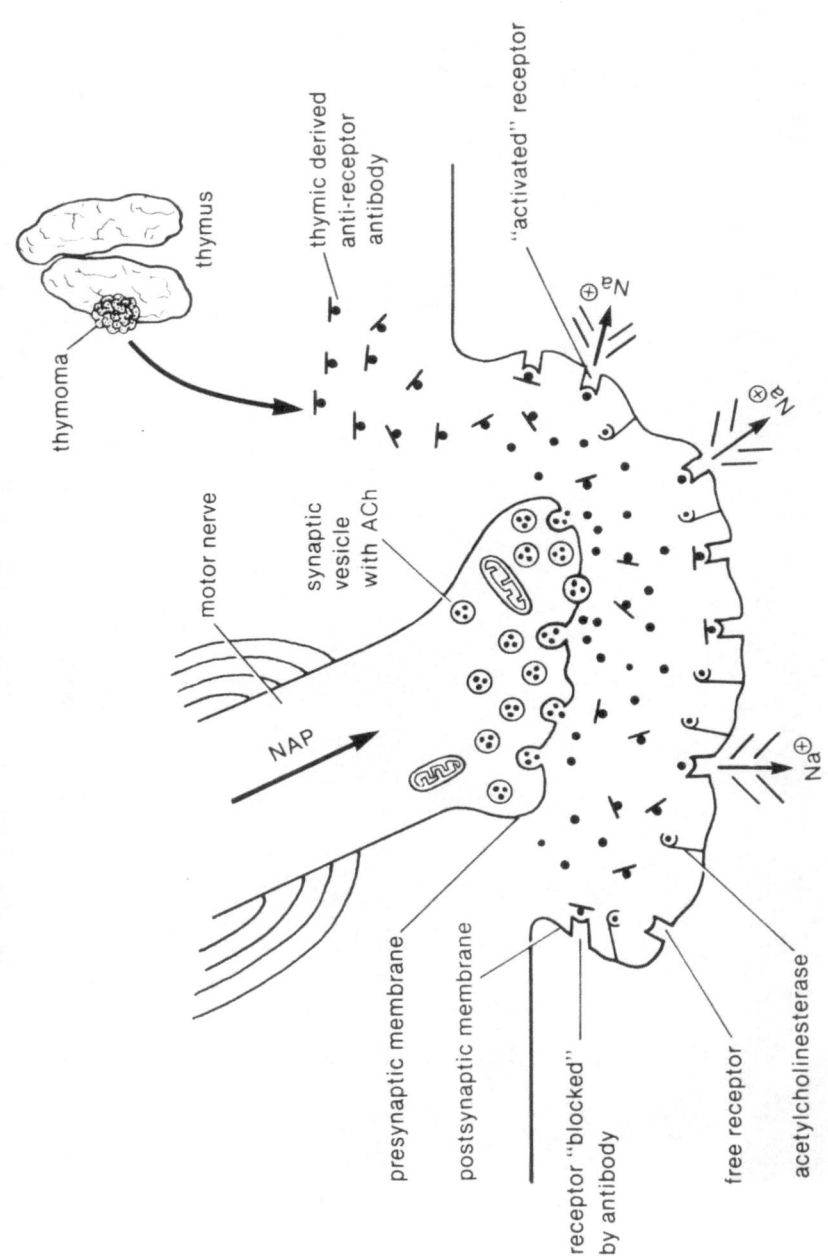

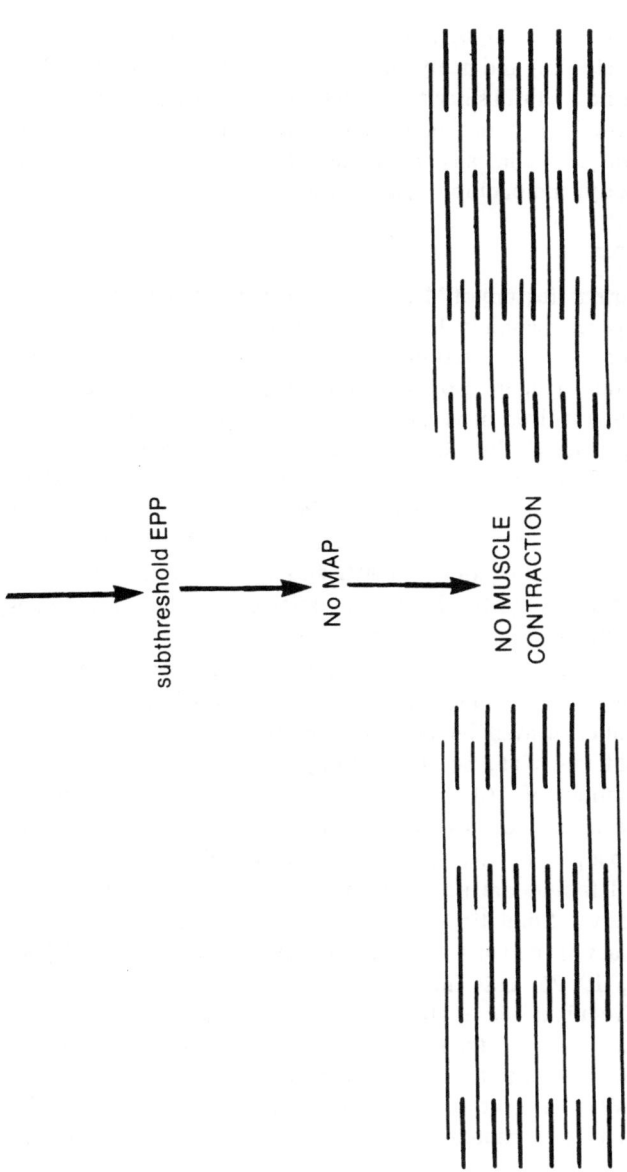

Figure 3-5. Diagrammatic representation of the pathophysiology in myasthenia gravis.

Laboratory Studies

The most useful laboratory studies for confirming the diagnosis of a suspected case of MG are the electromyogram (especially the repetitive nerve stimulation and single fiber studies) and acetylcholine receptor antibody (AChR-ab) titers. Muscle biopsy is not helpful since the muscle tissue is invariably normal in the disease. However, the biopsy may be of value when one is considering other neuromuscular diseases that clinically resemble MG (i.e., "ragged-red" fiber disease, myotonic atrophy, and oculopharyngeal muscular dystrophy).

Electrodiagnostic tests

The most characteristic feature of MG is neuromuscular fatigue. The electrical counterpart of this phenomenon is the progressive decline or decrement in the amplitude of the compound motor action potential to repetitive nerve stimulation at low and high rates (Figure 3-6). In any given patient with myasthenia, different muscles can be involved in varying degrees, and the presence of a normal response in a single muscle by no means excludes the diagnosis. A decremental response will be found in 70 to 85 percent of patients with generalized myasthenia if three or more muscles are tested. Proximal muscles such as the bicepts, deltoid or trapezius will frequently yield the best results. A decremental response, however, is not pathognomic of MG and can be seen in botulism, Eaton-Lambert syndrome, amyotropic lateral sclerosis, polio, myotonias, McArdle's disease, periodic paralysis and multiple sclerosis.

The phenomenon of decremental response results from progressive failure of more and more neuromuscular junctions in which transmission is precarious. At these sites, the number of available acetylcholine receptors is just sufficient to produce a threshold end plate potential (EPP). Thus the safety margin is reduced, and as the amount of ACh released declines with repetitive nerve stimulation (which is the normal occurrence), more and more junctions progressively fail. In normal people, the safety margin is sufficiently large so that decremental response and fatigue are not seen at rates of stimulation below 50/second. A modified nerve stimulation test has been described which may increase diagnostic accuracy in patients with mild localized or atypical MG (Desmedt and Borenstein, 1977). This double-step procedure combines forearm ischemia with repetitive ulnar nerve stimulation. A myasthenic patient typically develops a distinct decremental response under these condtions, whereas normal subjects maintain amplitude. A small percentage of patients with the clinical diagnosis of MG have normal repetitive nerve stimualtion studies. This group generally has a restricted form of disease in which only the lid and extraocular muscles are involved (ocular myasthenia). Since less than 20 percent of such patients show the decremental response, other procedures must be carried out to confirm the diagnosis. It is in this group of patients that

Technique:

1 Discontinue anticholinesterases (if possible) 24 hours prior to study
2 Immobilize limb to be studied and secure recording electrode (temperature of muscle tested should be 35 to 37°C)
3 Muscles to be studied:
   a. abductor digiti minimi (stimulate ulnar nerve)
   b. deltoid (stimulate axillary nerve)
   c. trapezius (stimulate accessory nerve)
4 Method of stimulation- stimulate at 3/second for two seconds with supramaximal stimulus (the decrement occurs in the first five responses so that six stimuli are sufficient).
5 The test is positive if the amplitude of the CMAP decrements by more than 10 percent.
6 If there is no significant decrement, exercise the muscle isometrically for 15 seconds and repeat step 4 immediately after exercise then exercise the muscle isometrically for 60 seconds and repeat step 4 at two to four minutes post-exercise (in some myasthenics the pre-exercise response is normal but the post-exercise phase is abnormal).
7 What should be seen in MG:

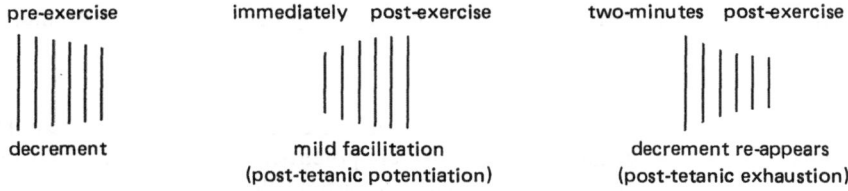

<table>
<tr><td>pre-exercise</td><td>immediately post-exercise</td><td>two-minutes post-exercise</td></tr>
<tr><td>decrement</td><td>mild facilitation
(post-tetanic potentiation)</td><td>decrement re-appears
(post-tetanic exhaustion)</td></tr>
</table>

8 If the study is normal, repeat study with muscles (b) and (c).

Figure 3-6. Repetitive nerve stimulation.

single fiber electromyography (SFEMG) is of value. Single fiber electromyography requires special equipment and skills. With this technique one can measure the variability of the time intervals between action potentials from pairs of muscle fibers belonging to the same motor unit. In myasthenia gravis this time interval (called jitter) is prolonged. Depending on the skills of the electromyographer as many as 75 percent of patients with ocular MG will have abnormal jitter.

Serologic tests

Acetylcholine receptor antibodies (AChR-ab) are found in the serum of over 90 percent of patients with myasthenia gravis. The majority of the approximate nine percent of patients who are diagnosed clinically as having MG but who lack AChR-ab in serum have a disease of recent onset, a non-autoimmune form of the disease (see Table 3-1), or purely ocular manifestations. Overall, 70 percent of ocular myasthenics will have elevated titers and this observation is useful (in combination with single fiber EMG) in confirming the diagnosis (Kelly et al, 1982). Since it is postulated that the antibody plays an important role in the pathogenesis of the disease, it is puzzling that the antibody titer frequently corresponds so poorly with the clinical severity of the disease. The discrepancy may be explained by the fact that the quantitative titer does not always reflect the functional activity of the antibodies (i.e., the ability of the antibody to block acetylcholine receptors and to accelerate their degradation) (Drachman et al, 1982).

A second serologic test that is of value is the anti-striational antibody titer. These antibodies are found in approximately 30 percent of MG patients and in 90 percent of patients with the disease who also have an associated thymoma. More recently, it has been demonstrated that patients with thymomas also have serum antibodies to an antigen (CAE) extracted by citric acid from skeletal muscle. The presence of CAE antibodies appears to be highly sensitive and specific for the detection of thymomas. In one study, ninety-five percent of myasthenics with these antibodies were found to have thymic tumors whereas the false positive and negative rates were very low (Gilhus et al, 1984). It is not known whether anti-striational antibodies have any pathogenic effect on muscle.

Pharmacologic tests

Pharmacologic tests including the use of endrophonium and curare are not of practical value for diagnosing MG. They are potentially hazardous and frequently give equivocal results. They are briefly discussed below.

1. Endrophonium test (see Figure 3-7): Edrophonium hydrochloride (Tensilon) is a short-acting anticholinesterase agent which is useful in the *management* of MG. Two mg. of the drug are injected intravenously and if there are no serious side effect (i.e., profound bradycardia), an additional 8 mg. are administered. A positive test means that there is significant clinical improvement in 10 to 30 seconds that wears off after five minutes. A positive test is suggestive of MG but may also be seen in Eaton-Lambert syndrome and botulism. A negative test (i.e., no clinical improvement) does not necessarily exclude MG especially if the disease is limited to the extraocular muscles. When administering the test it is wise to keep a syringe of atropine and Ambubag on hand in the event of the rare complication of cardiorespiratory collapse. During treatment, patients with myasthenia may become weaker. Often it is difficult to determine whether this increased disability is because of the myasthenia itself or is the result of overmedication (cholinergic crisis). The endrophonium test may be of value in such a situation. If the patient becomes weaker after receiving the drug, then he is probably overdosed. If, on the other hand, his strength improves, he is undermedicated. The danger of this test is that a given patient may be underdosed with respect to one muscle group and overdosed with respect to another. It would be a grave error to increase the dose of medication in a patient whose arms became stronger after edrophonium but whose respiratory function deteriorated. If the results of the test are equivocal, all medications should be with-

drawn. Such a patient should be placed in an intensive care setting where mechanical respirators are available. After several days of observation (drying out period), treatment is re-instituted as if this were a newly recognized case.

2. Curare test: The curare test can be used in patients whose clinical presentation is suggestive of MG but who have failed to demonstrate a decrement with the EMG study, and in situations where single fiber EMG and AchR-ab titers are not available. Myasthenics are 10 to 100 times more sensitive to the neuromuscular blocking effects of curare than are normals. This excessive sensitivity forms the basis for the diagnostic use of curare in the systemic and regional curare tests. Detailed measurements are made of the hand grips, ptosis, eye movements, head and leg holding against gravity, and vital capacity. One-tenth of the normal curarizing dose is given (16 mg/kg) intravenously with an anesthesiologist in attendance. A positve result consists of a clinically documented increase in the patient's weakness. In a normal person, such a small dose of curare has no effect. In myasthenics, however, even small amounts of this ACh-R blocker are sufficient to reduce the marginal end plate potentials below threshold. A safer variant of this test is the regional curare test.

Curare is injected distal to the placement of a blood pressure cuff applied to the arm to be tested. Repetitive nerve stimulation at 3/second is then performed with the cuff inflated (ischemic conditions) and after the cuff is released. A decrement of greater than ten percent is considered a positive test (Patten, 1978).

Treatment

To say merely that the treatment of myasthenia gravis is controversial is a gross understatement. Numerous reviews have been published regarding the management of this disorder with each group of authors proposing somewhat different formulas for successful therapy. Because controlled trials have not been done to evaluate the different treatment regimens comparatively, the choice of therapy remains somewhat arbitrary and subject to personal bias. The treatment discussed in the ensuing pages reflects the author's own personal bias. The reader is encouraged to review a recent publication by Rowland (1980) in which some of the more controversial issues regarding management of the myasthenic patient is addressed.

Successful management of myasthenia gravis begins with careful explanation of the disorder to the patient and family. A list of potentially hazardous medications should be provided. Such a list would include quinidine (and quinine in tonic water), propranolol, penicillamine (Aldrich et al, 1979), procainamide, and a variety of antibiotics (polymyxin, colistin, bacitracin, tetracyclines, and the "mycins" including kanamycin, neomycin, streptomycin, gentamycin) (Argov and Mastaglia, 1979). Patients should be warned that environmental

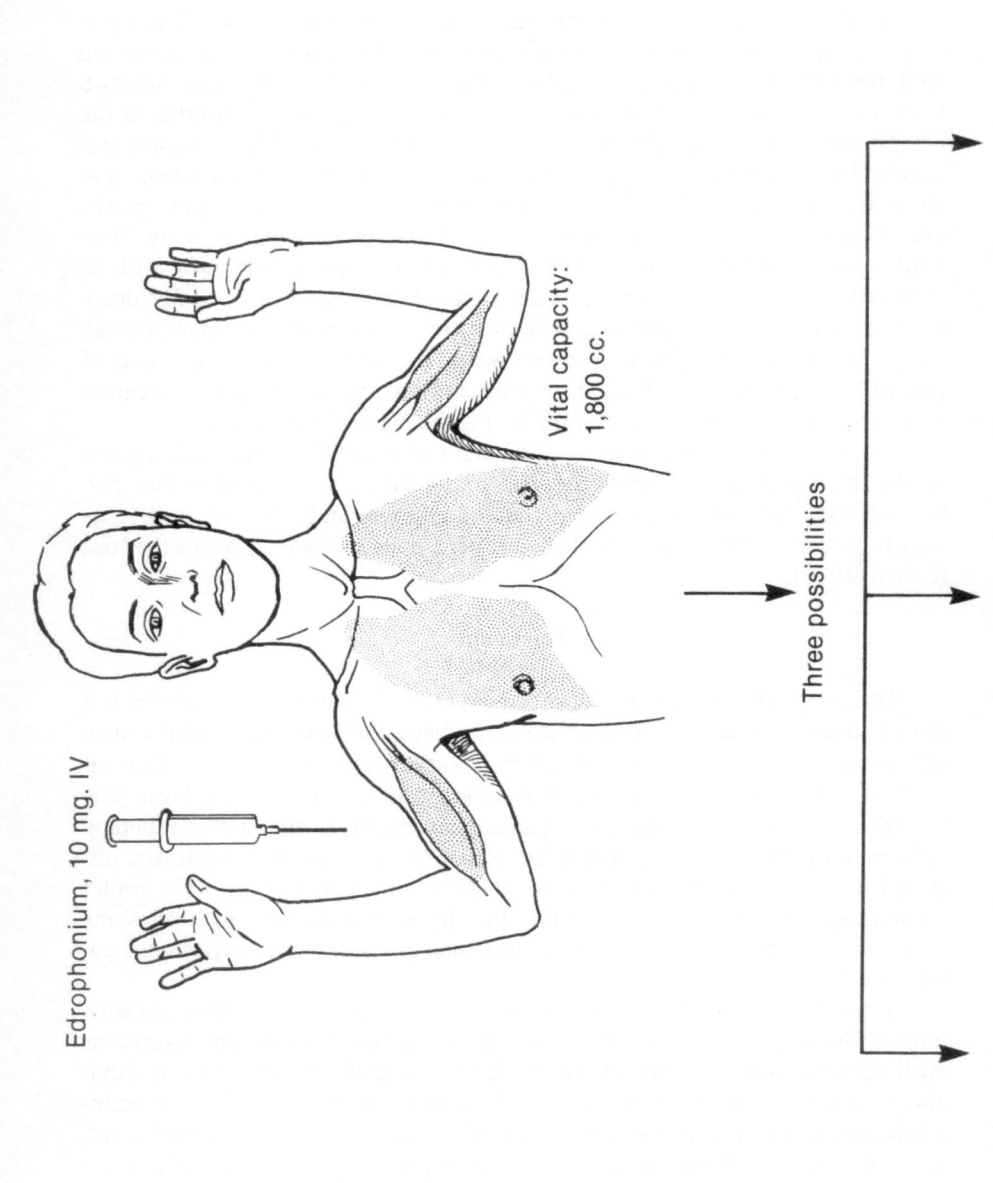

Edrophonium, 10 mg. IV

Vital capacity: 1,800 cc.

Three possibilities

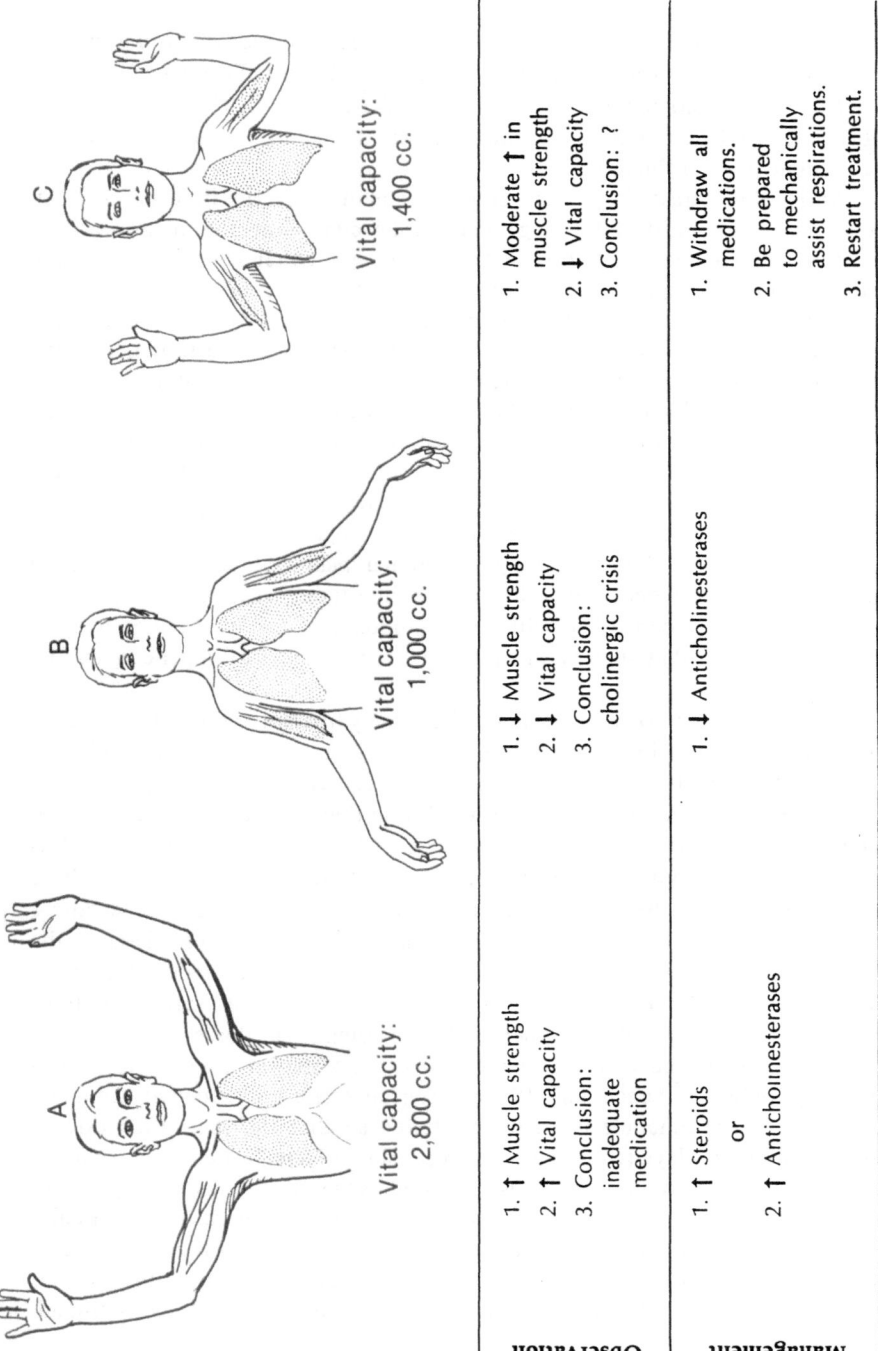

	A	B	C
Observation	Vital capacity: 2,800 cc.	Vital capacity: 1,000 cc.	Vital capacity: 1,400 cc.
	1. ↑ Muscle strength 2. ↑ Vital capacity 3. Conclusion: inadequate medication	1. ↓ Muscle strength 2. ↓ Vital capacity 3. Conclusion: cholinergic crisis	1. Moderate ↑ in muscle strength 2. ↓ Vital capacity 3. Conclusion: ?
Management	1. ↑ Steroids or 2. ↑ Antٖicholinesterases	1. ↓ Anticholinesterases	1. Withdraw all medications. 2. Be prepared to mechanically assist respirations. 3. Restart treatment.

Figure 3-7. The edrophonium test.

stresses such as extreme heat and emotional upset may exacerbate the disease. Pregnancy may also worsen the disease and certainly complicates management.

The pharmacologic approach to treating MG is twofold. One approach is to enhance transmission at the neuromuscular junction and the other is to suppress the immune basis of the disease.

Anticholinesterase drugs such as pyridostigmine are the first line of treatment. By temporarily inhibiting acetylcholinesterase at the neuromuscular junction they enhance the action of ACh at this site. Other agents such as guanidine, calcium, and ephedrine improve synaptic transmission by increasing the presynaptic relase of ACh and are much less effective in MG. Pyridostigmine is initiated at doses of 30-60 mg four times daily. The dose and time of administration are adjusted by trial and error to achieve maximum benefit. If the patient is having problems with weakness on awakening in the morning, the 180 mg. pyridostigmine timespan may be added at bedtime. It must be emphasized that the proper dose of anticholinesterases is whatever amount is needed to control symptoms. While most patients initially have an excellent clinical response to anticholinesterases, many become refractory to the medication and require progressively higher doses. Crampy abdominal pain and excessive salivation are common side effects of high dose anticholinesterase treatment. These symptoms can be easily controlled with small amounts of atropine but it is more important to note that such complaints are often warnings of impending cholinergic crisis.

Adrenocorticosteroids are beneficial in many patients with MG; however, the particular indications for the use of these agents have not been fully established. Oral prednisone is the agent of choice because it is inexpensive and effective. Furthermore, it has a short half-life so that alternate day therapy does not interfere with the pituitary-adrenal axis. All patients with generalized MG with or without thymomas are candidates for steroid treatment if they have been given an adequate trial of anticholinesterases and are still not leading a life that is satisfactory to them. Prior to the initiation of steroid therapy, the patient should be hospitalized and anticholinesterase doses reduced to their lowest obligatory levels (those that are necessary to maintain safe respirations and adequate swallowing). Treatment is begun using small doses of prednisone, 25 mg every day, and gradually increased by 12.5 mg increments every third dose (Seybould and Drachman, 1974). After adequate improvement has taken place, the dosage schedule is gradually altered so that the same total dose is given on alternate days (to minimize adverse side effects). When improvements have reached a maximum, the dose of prednisone can be lowered gradually over the course of the next several years (by 5 mg per month). Eventually, a maintenance level can be established but virtually all patients require indefinite continuation of steroids (Engel, 1976). With improvement of the patient, anticholinesterase medications can be further withdrawn and discontinued.

There are two major problems with prednisone therapy: side effects and the tendency for symptoms to recur as the steroid dose is tapered. In one study over thirty eight percent of myasthenic patients treated with steroids experienced serious side effects. Among the most frequent were weight gain, cataracts, diabetes mellitus, osteoporosis, diastolic hypertension, cardiac failure and gastric ulcertaion. Furthermore, only seven percent of the steroid treated patients were able to be completely withdrawn from the drug once it was initiated (Sghirlanzoni et al, 1984). Because of these problems thymectomy is the treatment of choice for all types of autoimmune MG except perhaps for those cases of restricted ocular myasthenia (Bever et al, 1983).

Thymectomy can be adequately accomplished only by splitting the sternum and thoroughly exploring the mediastinum. The transcervical approach is not suitable for this purpose.

Thymectomy may benefit myasthenics of either sex, with any severity or duration of illness. Cases of late-onset MG (i.e., symptoms beginning after age 55) may also benefit from the procedure even if upon removal of the tissue, the gland is found to be atrophic (Olanow et al, 1982). There is some evidence that when thymectomy is performed early in the course of the disease, the overall prognosis is better. However, because of the possibility of a spontaneous remission, this procedure should not be done earlier than six to twelve months after onset of the disorder (Drachman, 1978). Response to thymectomy cannot be predicted in individual cases, but overall 75 percent of patients improve, half of whom go into remission (Perlo et al, 1971). Some patients are markedly better a day or two following surgery, but in most cases, the response is delayed.

Patients who undergo thymectomy and were previously treated with steroids should receive corticosteroids prior to, during, and after surgery to prevent relative adrenal insufficiency, shock, and possibly death.

Thymectomy should be done on all patients who harbor a thymoma, for several reasons:

1. thirty-five percent of thymomas invade adjacent structures and may (rarely) metastasize to distance locales;
2. removal of the tumor is sometimes accompanied by significant improvement and even remission of myasthenia.

Therefore, initial evaluation of all new cases of MG should include a chest X-ray, tomograms and computed tomography (if available) of the anterior mediastinum as well as anti-striational antibody titers, to uncover such tumors. Computed tomography provides more information than plain radiographs or conventional tomography. It appears to be highly sensitive and specific for detecting thymomas in patients over the age of 40 years (Fon et al, 1982). Cor-

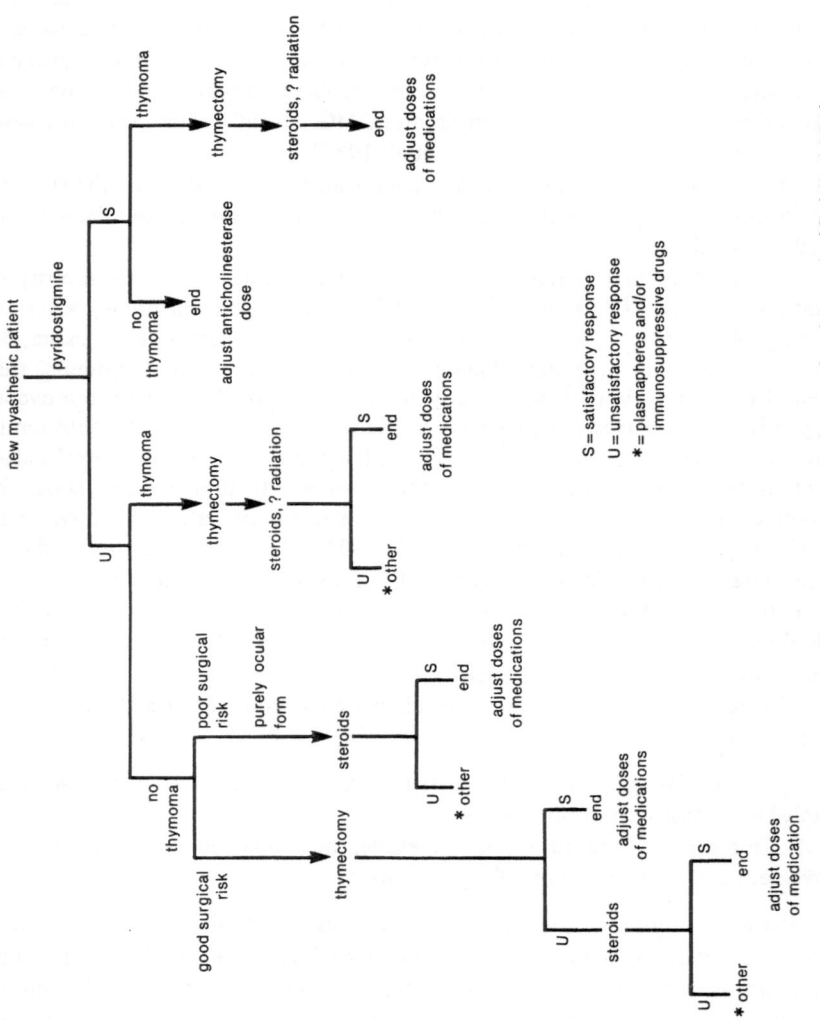

Figure 3-8. Summary of the management of myasthenia gravis (Galdi, 1978).

ticosteroid treatment is recommended after the removal of invasive thymomas and some believe that radiation therapy is also indicated in such instances. Plasmapheresis is a new weapon that has been added to the treatment arsenal. Because of the expense (over $800 per treatment), problems with availability, and complications (Rodnitzky and Goeken, 1982), plasmapheresis should be used only to get a patient out of a difficult period or in preparation for thymectomy. Frequently, immunosuppressive agents (azathioprine or cyclophosphamide) must be given in conjunction with the pheresis if more long term benefits are to be gained. An excellent review of this subject is provided by Dau (1980). The management of MG is outlined in Figure 3-8. An illustrative case history follows:

Case Report

A 26-year-old lady complained of fluctuating double vision. This was most troublesome when returning home after a long day of work. Often she found herself closing one eye, while driving, to eliminate the double image. In addition, she periodically noted difficulty in chewing and swallowing. Physical examination revealed bilateral mild ptosis, weakness in several extraocular muscles, palatal, jaw and neck flexor weakness. An edrophonium test was done and within 30 seconds of injecting the medication, her ptosis cleared and she hand increased palatal, jaw and neck flexor strength. There was no change in the ocular muscles. An EMG with repetitive nerve stimulation studies confirmed the diagnosis of myasthenia gravis. Anti-striational antibody titers as well as tomographic X-rays of the anterior mediastinum were obtained (both of which were normal) in order to evaluate the possibility of a thymoma. She was started on pyridostigmine 30 mg QID and initially did well. Over the next four months, increasing doses of pyridostigmine were need to maintain swallowing and chewing. When she was taking doses in excess of 150 mg, every three hours, stomach cramps and excessive salivation became prominent. Small doses of atropine alleviated these problems. One evening, extremely short of breath, she presented herself to the emergency room. In addition to generalized weakness, she was found to be hypoxic (arterial blood gas Pa O_2 50 mmHg) with a vital capacity of 700 ml. She then told the emergency room physician that she had increased her pyridostigmine dose without consulting a physician because she wanted to feel stronger. Ten milligrams of edrophonium were administered intravenously and a further decline in her vital capacity and peripheral strength was noted. She was felt to be in cholinergic crisis and was admitted to the intensive care unit where her respirations were mechanically supported. Anticholinesterases were witheld for 48 hours. She was then started on intramuscular pyridostigmine (0.5 mg every four hours). The dose was slowly increased over the next three days until she could sustain a vital capacity of 1500-2000 ml without mechanical assistance. She was then taken off the respiratory and switched to equivalent doses of oral pyridostigmine (1.0 mg intramuscular pyridostigmine = 30 mg oral pyrdostigmine).

One week later a thymectomy was performed and histologic examination of the gland revealed numerous islands of hyperplasia. She recovered uneventfully and left the hospital taking 30 to 60 mg of pyridostigmine every four hours. After doing well on this dose for several years, she once again began to require more frequent and greater amounts of medication to maintain adequate bulbar and limb strength (180 mg, every three to four hours). Examination carried out during the peak of her pyridostigmine dose (i.e. 1½ hours following p.o. administration) revealed significant weakness in many muscles and a vital capacity of 2200. Following the administration of 10 mg of intravenous edrophonium there was a slight increase in strength and vital capacity (2600 ml). It was decided to initiate steroid therapy and her pyridostigmine dose was decreased over the next three days to a level whereby she was just able to maintain adequate swallowing and a vital capcity of 1500.

Twenty-five milligrams of oral prednisone was administered daily and this dose was increased by 12.5 mg increments every third day. When her daily prednisone dose reached 50 mg she noted marked improvement in her strength. Vital capacity at this time measured 2900 ml. Over the next 20 days, her prednisone dose was altered so that at the end of this period she was receiving 100 mg every other day (see schedule):

Day	Prednisone dose (mg)	Day	Prednisone dose (mg)
0	50	11	20
1	45	12	80
2	55	13	15
3	40	14	85
4	60	15	10
5	35	16	90
6	65	17	5
7	30	18	95
8	70	19	0
9	25	20	100
10	75		

She left the hospital with excellent functional strength and vital capacity (3600 ml). She did well, and after two months found that she required only 30 mg of pyridostigmine twice per day. It was decided to taper her prednisone by 5 mg decrements every four weeks. Following this regimen she was able to reduce her prednisone to 20 mg every other day. However, she found that further decrements resulted in significant loss of strength. Because of this, she is currently maintained on 30 mg of prednisone on alternate days. The plan is to decrease her prednisone at a slower pace (i.e., by 2.0 mg every 4 weeks).

CHAPTER 4

The Muscular Dystrophies

SEVERE X-LINKED RECESSIVE MUSCULAR DYSTROPY (DUCHENNE-TYPE)

The best known and most frequently encountered of the dystrophies is the severe X-linked recessive variety. Initially described in 1868 by Guillaume Duchenne, the disease is characterized by rapidly progressive generalized muscle weakness and "pseudohypertrophy" of certain muscle groups. Death during the 2nd or 3rd decade is the inevitable outcome in all cases. Duchenne muscular dystropy (DMD) is not an uncommon disorder. From 20 to 33 cases per 100,000 live male births are reported annually. Since the disease is inherited in an X-linked recessive manner, one-half of the male offspring of a relatively unaffected mother (carrier) will manifest the illness. Previously it was believed that up to one-third of cases resulted from spontaneous mutation either in the patient or his mother. However, with improved methods of carrier detection, it appears that such mutations are relatively uncommon.

It is known that some X-linked recessive disorders can manifest in females with normal karyotypes by inactivation of the paternal X-chromosome or lyonization. Despite this, Duchenne's dystrophy in females of normal karyotype is a rare event. Most female carriers are asymptomatic or have minimal non-progressive weakness. However, the typical clinical and laboratory features of Duchenne dystrophy have been described in a 9-year-old girl who appeared to be a manifesting heterozygote (Gomez et al, 1977). Her identical twin was normal, but the mother's brother had DMD and both the mother and the twin sister in question were identified as carriers by CPK tests. An additional case of a young girl with progressive muscle disease in a family with an extensive history of DMD has been reported by Olson and Fenichel (1982).

Clinical Presentation: Signs and Symptoms

The infant with Duchenne's dystrophy attains all the early motor milestones on time and initially appears quite normal. Lack of apparent abnormalities in the earlier periods is probably due to the crudity of our observations. At about age 2½ however, it becomes obvious that there is something wrong with the child. He is observed to walk with his heels slightly raised off the ground and he is unable to keep pace with his peers. Falls are common, and the child is seen to rise from the floor by placing his hands on his knees and virtually "walking" his hands up his thighs (Gowers' sign). By age three or four waddling, lordotic gait is noted, and the child complains of difficulty climbing stairs and rising from a seated position. As the strength of the normal child increases, so the strength of some Duchenne patients may appear to increase up to the age of ten, only to decline later. With time, progressive disability ensues so that in most cases by the end of the first decade, there is generalized muscle weakness and wasting (with sparing of the bulbar structures) and a wheelchair is required. Once the wheelchair is used, kyphoscoliosis and fixed joint contractures are likely to occur. Obesity, impaired circulation to the lower extremities with dependent edema, and mental and emotional problems are further complications of a wheelchair existence. Recurrent pulmonary infections secondary to mechanically impaired ventilatory effort are common at this stage. By the end of the second decade, the majority of patients have succumbed to pneumonia and/or cardiac disease.

Muscle pseudohypertrophy is seen in 85 to 90 percent of cases. This varies from minor degrees of muscle enlargement to gross hypertrophy. When present, it is most commonly seen in the calves, but it may involve the quadriceps muscle and shoulder and hip girdle musculature as well.

Many of the affected boys are mentally dull and almost 30 percent have IQs under 75 (Poser et al, 1969). This mental subnormality is present from birth and is nonprogressive.

Although the heart at autopsy frequently shows extensive damage, symptoms of congestive heart failure are surprisingly uncommon in Duchenne's dystrophy. Electrocardiographic evidence of myocardial dysfunction is noted at an early stage, and includes tall R waves in the right precordial leads (V1 and V2) and deep Q waves in the left precordial leads (V5 and V6). Lethal arrhythmias may occur. Echocardiography frequently reveals contraction abnormalities in the left ventricular wall (Goldberg et al, 1982).

Laboratory Studies

While cases of DMD can frequently be recognized on the basis of the patient's history and clinical signs, further laboratory evaluation is mandatory to confirm the diagnosis. Other neuromuscular disorders may be confused with DMD, and while it would not be catastrophic to mistake a case of spinal muscular atrophy for DMD, it would certainly be tragic to have missed treatable entities such as polymyositis and muscle carnitine deficiency. Definite diagnosis is also needed for prognostication and proper genetic counseling.

Serum muscle enzymes

Extremely high levels of creatine phosphokinase (in the thousands) are frequently found in the early stages of Duchenne's dystrophy. Such elevations are usually present from birth and precede evidence of clinical involvement. Elevations of muscle enzymes to such degrees are rarely, if every, seen in the spinal muscular atrophies. As the disease progresses, CPK values fall, but never reach normal values.

Electromyography

The most commonly observed EMG abnormality in Duchenne's dystrophy is the "BSAPP" pattern. This consists of short duration (brief), low amplitude (small), numerous for the amount of force called on to produce (abundant), polyphasic potentials. Fibrillations may also be seen.

Muscle biopsy

Muscle biopsy must be done in all suspected cases in order to rule out other more treatable myopathies (i.e., muscle carnitine deficiency and polymyositis) that may mimic the dystrophies. The histologic abnormalities of dystrophic muscle are similar whatever the specific category. Under the light miscroscope, there is variation in fiber size with small rounded fibers adjacent to extremely large ones. Necrotic fibers are abundant. The origin of the hypertrophied fibers is uncertain but they could be explained by the hypertrophy of relative normal fibers compensating for damaged ones. As the disease progresses, there is proliferation of endomysial and perimysial connective tissue and fat. A variable inflammatory response with phagocytosis of fibers may also be seen (see Figure 4-1). Because patients with DMD may be at risk for anesthetic induced malignant hyperthermia, muscle biopsies should be performed using only *local* anesthetics. The muscle tissue excised should be evaluated to determine susceptibility to malignant hyperthermia (see Chapter 5).

Pathogenesis

Currently there are three main theories regarding the pathogenesis of the muscular dystrophies:

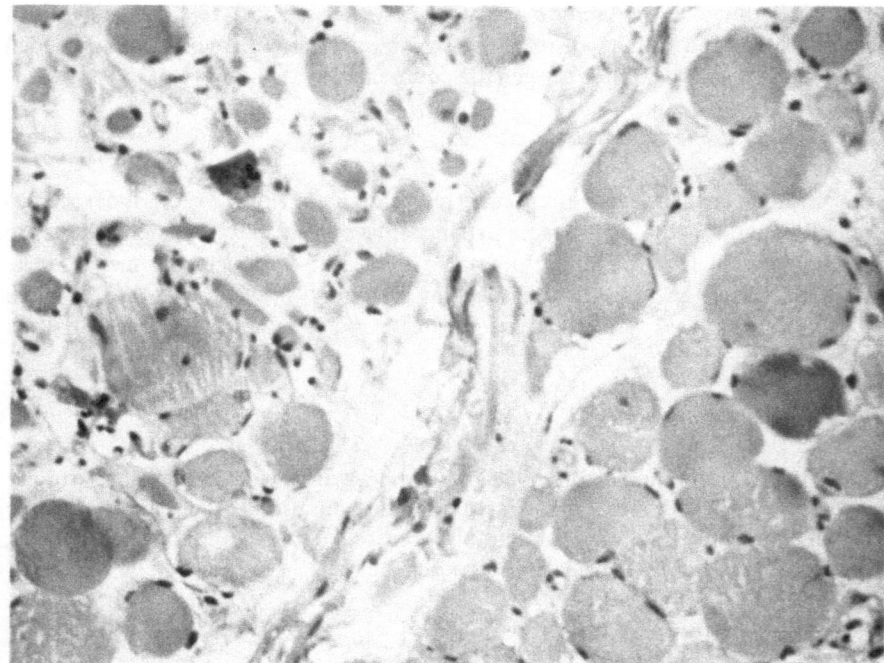

Figure 4-1. Muscle biopsy—Duchenne's dystrophy. Note the variation in fiber size, the increased endomysial connective tissue, and the phasocytosis of degenerating fibers.

Vascular theory

This theory, which suggest that inadequate blood flow might account for the degeneration of dystrophic muscle tissue, received its support from the work of Demos (1961) who found slowed arm-to-tongue circulation time in patients and in carriers of Duchenne dystrophy. Other evidence favoring a vascular origin is the observation that groups of necrotic fibers suggesting microinfarcts are seen early in the disease, and similar lesions can be produced in rats by embolization (Hathaway et al, 1970). However, morphological similarity between dystrophies and experimental myopathies does not necessarily prove an identical etiology. Furthermore, more recent studies of blood flow in dystrophic muscle have failed to demonstrate any abnormality (Paulson et al, 1974).

Neurogenic theory

Proponents of this theory believe that the dystrophies result from disordered neural influences on the muscle. In support of this theory is the observation that muscle taken from dystrophic patients and grown in culture (and therefore deprived of neural input) fails to reproduce the morphologic abnormalities characteristic of the disease (Bishop et al, 1971). Cardiac involvement speaks against the neural hypothesis.

Membrane theory

To date, the most widely accepted theory as to the pathogenesis of Duchenne's dystrophy attributes the disease to abnormal membrane function. Genetic mutations could result in such missing or structurally altered membrane proteins that the membrane becomes unusually permeable and cannot maintain the required internal milieu for proper cell function (Rowland, 1980). Evidence for this hypothesis, however, is at best circumstantial. Abnormal behavior of some of the enzymes associated with the sarcolemmal and erythrocyte cell membranes has been noted (Brown et al, 1967), but the significance of these findings is still uncertain. Electrophysiologic studies on DMD and control muscle grown in culture have failed to substantiate any physiologic difference between the membranes of these tissues (Rothman and Bischoff, 1983).

More recently, it has been suggested that the disease may result from loss of genetic control of muscle proteolytic enzymes. Normally these enzymes are involved in the physiologic turnover of muscle proteins. However, in dystrophic muscles, these enzymes are found to have increased activity which may account for the excessive fiber destruction.

Treatment

Various agents including steroids, allopurinol, plant growth stimulants, leucine and proteinase inhibitors have been used as treatment in the dystrophies without succes. However, much can be done to make the life of the patient more comfortable. As discussed by Siegel (1978), therapy should be administered by a team that includes the pediatrician along with neurologic, orthopedic, genetic and physiatric consultants. The primary physician should be in charge of coordinating all consulting activities. He should arrange for the patient to be seen by a neurologist three or four times per year for periodic measurement of strength and function. Such measurement is essential in the management of activity and exercise, and in the proper timing of psychiatric, orthotic, and surgical treatment.

Physical therapy should be organized with each visit to the neurologist and the patient should be encouraged to continue the therapy at home. Passive tendon stretching combined with active exercise to increase strength in healthy muscles effectively retards the natural progression of joint contractures. When indicated, orthopedic consultants may be called upon to evalute the need for surgical procedures, including correction of contractures, bracing, heel-cord lengthening, and tendon transfers, all of which have proved successful in maintaining mobility. The additional period of ambulation afforded by such procedures may represent up to 20 percent of the patient's life span and thus provides an important benefit (Vignos et al, 1963). Because dystrophic patients frequently have inadquate pulmonary reserve, they are particularly liable to respiratory failure when exposed to depressant drugs. For this reason, the anesthesiologist must carefully monitor the cardiorespiratory status of the patient during such surgical procedures.

Cardiomyopathy is a complication of all forms of muscular dystrophy. However, relatively few patients show overt clinical evidence of heart disease until late in their course. Serial chest x-rays, electrocardiograms, and pulmonary function studies are mandatory. Treatment of congestive heart failure and/or arrhythmias should be promptly instituted. In addition, the patient should be instructed on the principles of pulmonary hygiene and chest therapy.

Genetic Counselling and Carrier Detection

Because no effective treatment is currently available, genetic counselling is extremely important. The primary purpose is to provide accurate information to the parents about the risk that any of their children may inherit the muscular dystrophy gene. Such counselling depends upon the identification of potential carriers of the disease which includes the patient's mother, sisters, and maternal aunts. When a woman who is a known carrier of the gene for DMD is pregnant, there are four possible outcomes. One-half of her female offspring will be carriers, and one-half of her sons will have the disease. The remaining siblings will be genetically and clinically normal. At the present time, the most reliable method of carrier detection is serum creatine phosphokinase (CPK) determination. Elevated CPK levels are found in 60 to 80 percent of heterozygotes (Hughes et al, 1971). Therefore, a normal level is not conclusive evidence against the carrier state. Additional information can be obtained by testing the subject's daughters and sisters. However, when evaluating CPK levels in females, one must take into account that CPK activity normally declines as sexual maturity is attained and rises again as the menopause is reached. For this reason, young sisters of affected boys should have their CPK levels measured as soon as possible and the physician should not wait until the girls "grow up." Some women may decide to have the sex of the fetus determined (by amniocentisis) during the 13th to 15th week of pregnancy with the intention of terminating the pregnancy if the fetus is male.

It would be preferable to identify afflicted males in utero so that normal male fetuses could be spared. This has not been possible to date.

In some instances, physical examination of potential carriers may unmask the heterozygous state. A variable percent age of such individuals (up to 80 percent in one study) (Roses et al, 1976) may have demonstrable proximal muscle weakness and/or hypertrophic muscles.

Other possible screening procedures for carrier identification include (1) serum pyruvate kinase determination (Percy et al, 1979), (2) serum hemopexin levels (Danieli and Angelini, 1976), (3) serum LDH isoenzyme patterns (Roses et al, 1977), (4) muscle biopsy (Roy and Dubowitz, 1970), and (5) erythrocyte studies (Percy and Miller, 1975; Miller et al, 1976).

BENIGN X-LINKED RECESSIVE MUSCULAR DYSTROPHY (BECKER TYPE)

Since Becker and Keiner's initial descritpion in 1955 of a slowly progressive variant of X-linked recessive muscular dystrophy, numerous families with this syndrome have been reported. Apart from the later onset and prolonged course, the clinical characteristics of this form of dystrophy (Becker's dystrophy) closely resemble those seen in the Duchenne type. Common to both are (1) onset with affliction of the pelvofemoral muscles, (2) pseudohypertrophy of the calves, and (3) involvement of the upper limbs in the later stages.

Both the Becker and Duchenne types are inherited in an X-linked recessive manner. However, linkage studies indicate that the genes probably occur at different loci on the X-chromosome (Skinner et al, 1974).

Clinical Presentation: Signs and Symptoms

There is a considerable range of clinical severity with the benign X-linked dystrophies. However, cases within families generally tend to follow a similar course. Symptoms generally appear in patients between the ages of 3 and 21 years (mean age of onset, 11 years) with initial complaints of difficulty with walking and mounting stairs. This reflects weakness of the quadriceps, hip extensors, and flexors. Later, tibialis anterior weakness and foot drop may develop.

Disease progression is slow, so that very few patients are unable to walk prior to age 25. The mean age for loss of ambulation is about 35 years (Bradley et al, 1978). Muscle hypertrophy is a common early manifestation and usually includes the calves and forearm musculature (see Figure 4-2). Weakness of the upper limbs inevitably occurs. However, two to fifteen years may elapse from the onset of lower extremity paresis before such involvement becomes ap-

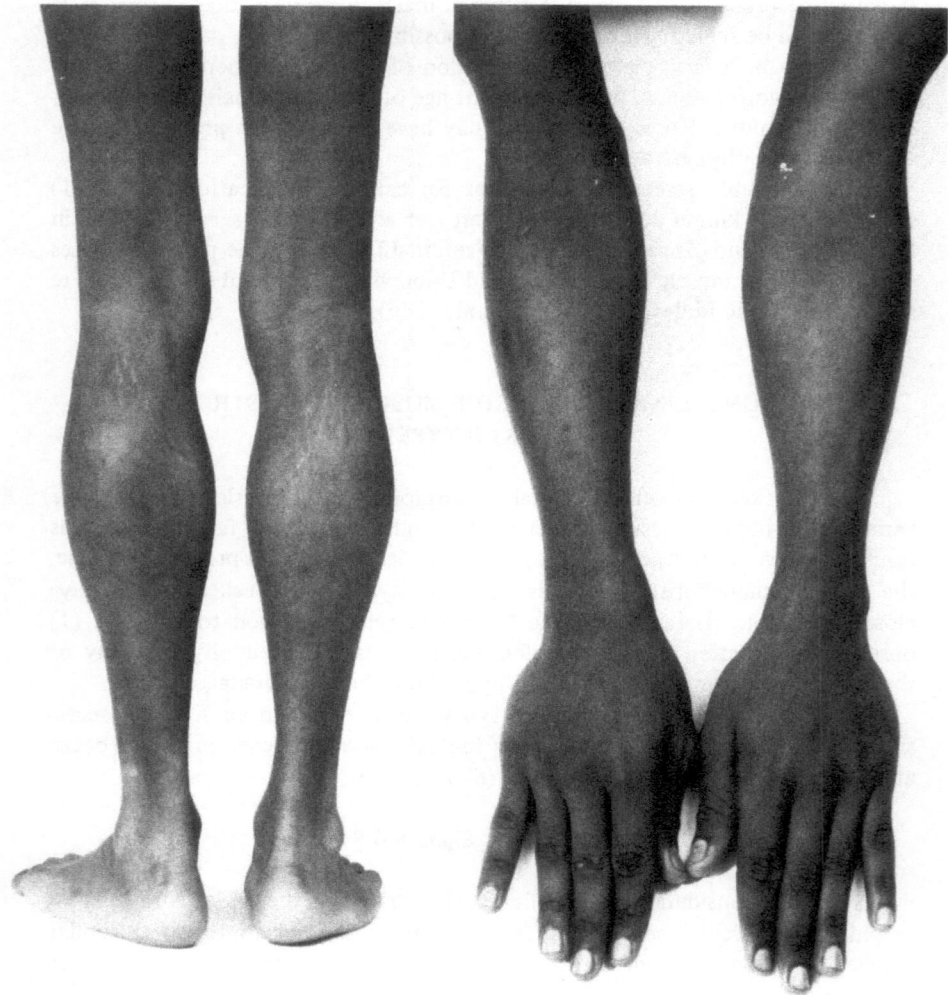

Figure 4-2. Becker dystrophy. Note the relative hyperliophy of the calves and forearms.

parent. Pectoralis major, serratus anterior, biceps, and brachioradialis are the earliest and most severely involved of the upper limb musculature. Cranial musculature is generally spared. For some patients, life expectancy is reduced, though others have survived into the 7th decade with the disease.

Mental retardation is much less common in comparison with Duchenne's dystrophy and is found in less than 15 percent of patients. It is never severe.

Although electrocardiographic abnormalities are present in almost half the patients with Becker dystrophy, clinical cardiac disease is unusual. Flattened or inverted T waves, elevated S-T segments, and prominent right precordial R waves have been described (Markand et al, 1969). Recently, a family has been reported (Kuhn et al, 1979) with severe cardiac involvement complicating their form of Becker's dystrophy, and with death from congestive heart failure occurring at an early age in one family member.

In summary, the clinical criteria for the diagnosis of Becker's dystrophy include (1) X-linked recessive inheritance, (2) ambulation maintained at least until age 16, (3) muscle pseudohypertrophy, and (4) specific distribution of muscle weakness and wasting involving the hip girdle and proximal lower extremities early, and the shoulder girdle and proximal upper limbs at a later stage.

Laboratory Studies

Muscle enzymes

Serum muscle enzymes including creatine phosphokinase and aldohase are elevated four to fortyfold in most patients with the disease. With age, the CPK levels tend to decrease, but they are never normal.

Electrodiagnostic testing

At rest, the muscles of dystrophic patients frequently show fibrillation potentials and positive sharp waves. When the muscle is called upon to produce joint movement, small, brief polyphasic motor units are seen.

Muscle biopsy

On the basis of muscle histology alone it is difficult to distinguish Becker's dystrophy from other slowly progressive neuromuscular diseases. Most commonly, the biopsy from such patients demonstrates fiber hypertrophy and atrophy (variation in fiber size), fiber splitting, increased numbers of internal nuclei, pyknotic nuclear clumps, areas of focal necrosis, and numerous regenerating fibers. In addition, marked endomysial connective tissue proliferation is generally apparent.

Treatment and Carrier Detection

There is no specific therapy for Becker's dystrophy and because of this, genetic counselling and carrier detection are of utmost importance. Approximately 50 percent of definite carriers (defined as a daughter of an affected man or a woman with an affected son and who comes from a family with a history of other male relatives similarly affected), have elevated CPK levels (Emery et al, 1967). In addition, judicious manual muscle testing may reveal significant weakness in a high proportion of femal heterozygotes (Ross et al, 1977).

BENIGN X-LINKED MUSCULAR DYSTROPHY
(EMERY-DREIFUSS TYPE)

Emery-Dreifuss dystrophy is a form of dystrophy manifested by weakness and wasting in a humeroperoneal distribution, early contractures, and cardiac disease. It is a rare disorder which prior to the report of Hopkins et al (1981) had been described in only six families.

Clinical Presentation: Signs and Symptoms

Symptoms of the disease begin in the upper limbs between the ages of two and ten years. Early in the course, there are contractures of the elbows and posterior cervical muscles. Weakness is initially confined to the bicep and tricep muscles with involvement later of the distal leg musculature. The disease is slowly progressive, and after age twenty appears to stabilize. Most patients remain ambulatory. Muscle hypertrophy, so characteristic of the Duchenne and Becker varieties of X-linked dystrophies, does not occur. Cranial musculature is seldom if ever involved.

A consistent feature of the disease is the cardiac conduction abnormality. Electrocardiograms reveal varying degrees of atrioventricular block, and patients may suffer from recurrent episodes of syncope, cerebral emboli and stroke.

Emery-Dreifuss dystrophy differs in so many ways from the Duchenne and Becker types that it should not be confused with these disorders. The prominent weakness and contractures of the arms, the absence of calf hypertrophy, and the cardiac conduction problems are distinctive features of Emery-Dreifuss dystrophy. Its X-linked mode of inheritance and the absence of cranial musculature involvement distinguish it from other varieties of muscular dystrophy (i.e., facioscapulohumeral and scapuloperoneal varieties).

Laboratory Studies

Muscle enzymes

The creatine phosphokinase levels are elevated in Emery-Dreifuss dystrophy but not to the magnitude seen in Duchenne's or Becker's dystrophies.

Electrodiagnostic tests/muscle biopsy

While the disease is characterized by stereotyped clinical manifestations, its electromyographic and pathological characteristics are somewhat variable. The EMG may have neurogenic, "myopathic", or mixed features. In most cases, the biopsy shows the characteristic changes of the dystrophies (i.e., fiber size variability, necrotic fibers, increased numbers of fibers with internal nuclei, fiber splitting, and increased endomysial connective tissue) but in some instances, neurogenic features are prominent. Whether the disease is truly a primary myopathy or a form of spinal muscular atrophy is probably of little significance (see discussion of Rowland et al, 1979).

Treatment

Treatment of the disorder is aimed at correction of the contractures and of cardiac conduction defects. Surgical release of the joint contractures provides the patient with greater ease and range of movement. Cardiac evaluation for insertion of a demand pacemaker is mandatory for all patients.

OCULOPHARYNGEAL DYSTROPHY

Slowly progressive ophthalmoplegia, later complicated by facial, pharyngeal, and limb weakness characterizes the clinical course of oculopharyngeal dystrophy. In approximately 50 percent of cases the condition is familial, with autosomal dominant inheritance being the most frequently observed pattern. While the illness is rare in most parts of the world, it is common among the French-Canadian families of Quebec and Spanish-American families in the southwestern sectors of the United States.

Clinical Presentation: Signs and Symptoms

Typically, the dystrophic process begins in the 4th decade with ptosis being the most common initial manifestation. Cases having their onset in childhood have been reported (Mathew et al, 1970). In some patients, the ptosis may be followed by progressive limitation of ocular movements leading to total ophthalmoplegia. However, many patients do not develop any weakness of the extraocular muscles other than in the lid elevators. The pupils are always spared. With the passage of time, the muscles of facial expression, mastication, and swallowing are affected. Esophageal motility studies indicate that the abnormal pharyngeal contractility is not confined to the striated muscle, but involves the smooth muscle as well. In some families, prominent proximal or distal limb weakness is part of the syndrome (Satoyoshi and Kinoshita, 1977). Many years may pass from the time of onset of the ocular symptoms to evidence of involvement elsewhere. Life expectancy may be shortened by the disease with aspiration pneumonia and/or emaciation being the most common causes of early demise.

Non-familial cases of oculopharyngeal dystrophy (OPD) may superficially resemble a number of neuromuscular disorders including myasthenia gravis, myotonic atrophy, "ragged-red" fiber disease, and polymyositis. Distinguishing OPD from myasthenia may be troublesome because besides their obvious clinical similarities, both are characterized pharmacologically by increased sensitivity to d-tubocurare (Ross, 1963). However, OPD has none of the volatile remitting or exacerbating qualities of myasthenia gravis. Furthermore, myasthenia is distinguished electrically by the characteristic decrement in the amplitude of the compound motor action potential with repetitive stimulation, which is corrected by anticholinesterase drugs (i.e., edrophonium).

Because of the prominent ptosis accompanied, in some instances, by distal weakness, OPD may be confused with myotonic atrophy. However, the frontal balding, cataracts, endocrine and ECG abnormalities, so prominent in the latter, are never seen in OPD. Furthermore, electrical myotonia is not found in OPD.

The absence of "ragged-red" fibers on the muscle biopsy, the normal CSF protein, and ECG help in differentiating cases of oculocraniosomatic neuromuscular disease from OPD. Polymyositis may be erroneously diagnosed in patients with OPD because of the strong inflammatory response in some of the biopsies of the latter (Bosch, et al, 1979). However, other histologic features characteristic of myositis are not evident. In addition, prominent ocular involvement is rarely encountered in cases of myositis.

Laboratory Studies

Serum muscle enzymes

Serum muscle enzyme levels, including CPK, are normal or mildly elevated in patients with OPD.

Electrodiagnostic studies

Repetitive nerve stimulation must be done in all suspected cases of OPD in order to distinguish it from myasthenia gravis. The decremental response which is characteristic of the latter has never been reported in a case of OPD.

Needle electromyography of involved muscles in OPD most commonly shows a "BSAPP" pattern.

Muscle biopsy

Variability of fiber size, increased internal nuclei, and moth-eaten fibers are nonspecific abnormalities seen in the muscle tissue of patients with OPD. In addition, shaply punched out, rimmed vacuoles occur in numerous fibers, and although these vacuoles are not specific for OPD, they are more abundant in this disorder than in any other neuromuscular disease (Brooke, 1973).

Other changes such as fibrosis and phagocytosis that are ordinarily considered hallmarks of the dystrophies, are not commonly seen in OPD.

Pathophysiology

It is now clear that patients with OPD suffer from a dystrophic process and not from a form of degenerative motor neuron disease as was once believed. Autopsy studies of such patients reveal no evidence of cranial nerve or anterior horn cell abnormalities (Schwarz and Liu, 1954; Satoyoshi and Kinoshita, 1977). Myopathic changes in the muscle constitute the predominant pathologic findings.

Treatment

There is no specific treatment of OPD. Supportive care, including surgical lifting of the lids to improve the ptosis, and insertion of a feeding gastrostomy tube to maintain adequate nutrition, greatly improve the patient's quality of life. Regular physiotherapy is also helpful in patients with significant limb involvement in order to prevent contractures and disuse atrophy.

FACIOSCAPULOHUMERAL DYSTROPHY

Facioscapulohumeral (FSH) dystrophy is a familial neuromuscular disorder usually transmitted in an autosomal dominant fashion. The clinical distribution of the muscle weakness and wasting is concentrated about the areas indicated by the descriptive title (i.e., facial muscles, muscles attached to the scapulae, and to a lesser extent, the proximal upper extremities).

Characteristic of the disease is its variable expression from family to family and within families as well. There may be severe, mild, and abortive forms amongst siblings of common parents.

As with the other dystrophies, the pathogenesis of the disease at the present time is uncertain.

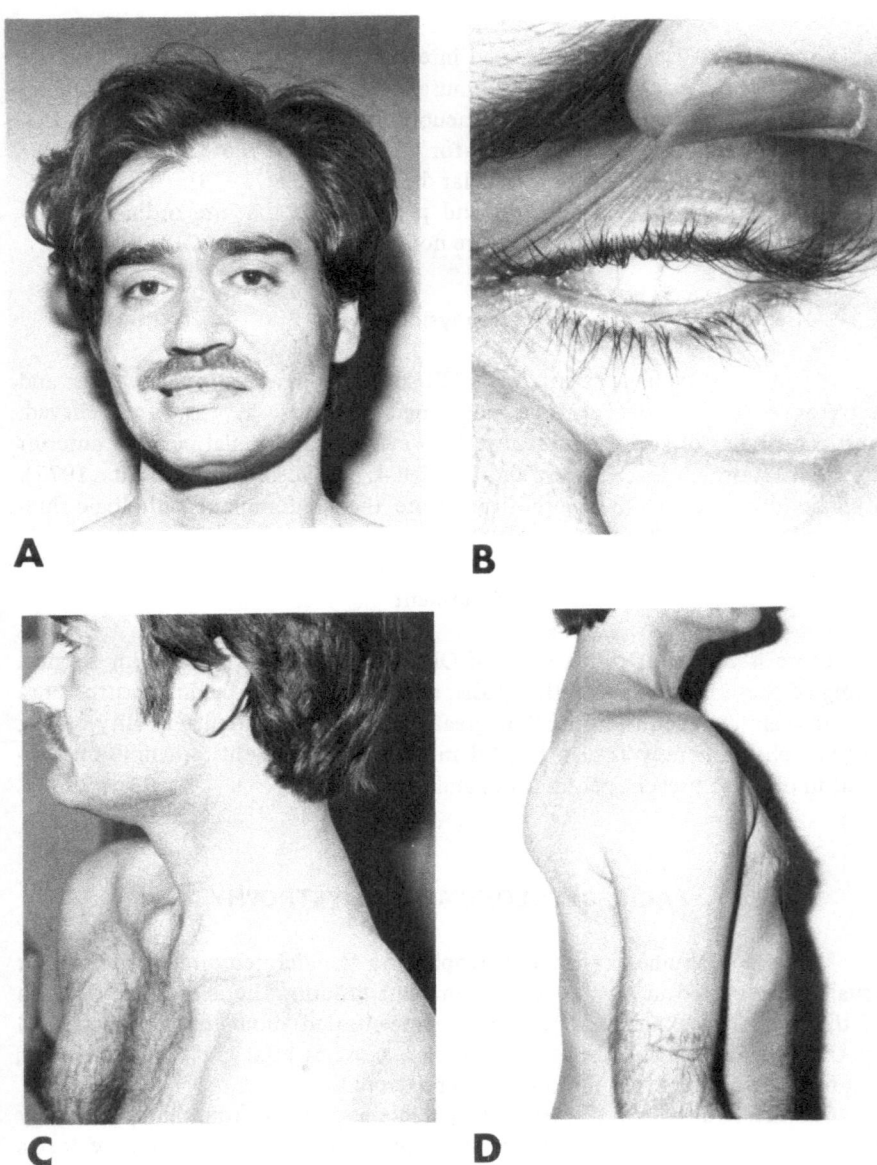

Figure 4-3. Note the weakness of the facial muscles and the inability of the patient to fully retract the corners of the mouth (A) or maintain eye closure against resistance (B). Atrophy of the neck muscles, upper arms, and shoulder girdle are demonstrated in C, D, and E. Note how the scapulae rise over the upper borders of the trapezius with attempted abduction of the arms (F).

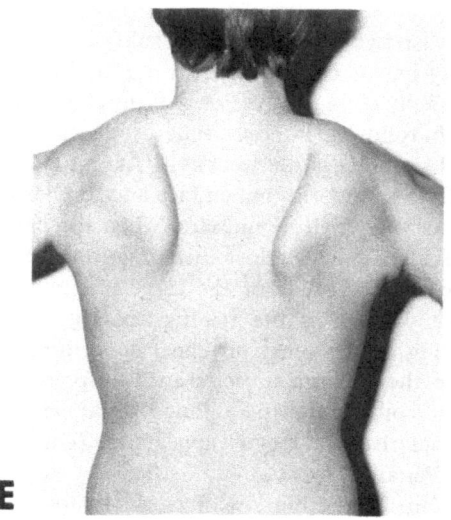

E

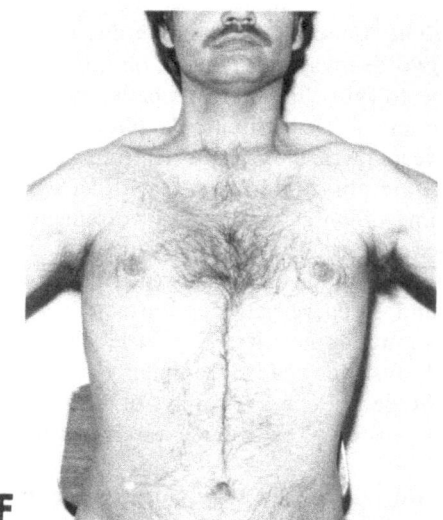

F

Clinical Presentation: Signs and Symptoms

There exist at least two distinct clinical subtypes of FSH dystrophy. The more common variety has its onset in the second or third decade. Facial weakness with inability to fully close the eyes or puff the cheeks is typically the initial manifestation. This is followed in short time by the development of proximal upper extremity and shoulder girdle weakness. At this stage in the disease, the patient is noted to have a smooth unlined face and forehead and atrophy of the neck, upper arm and shoulder girdle muscles. When the patient attempts to abduct the arms, the scapulae, having lost their fixation, are seen riding over the back and above the upper border of the trapezius muscles (see Figure 4-3). Characteristic of the disorder is the relative sparing of the deltoid muscles despite marked wasting of the other proximal upper limb muscles (i.e., biceps and triceps). Because the forearm muscles are well preserved, they appear unusually prominent in contrast to the thinned proximal structures. This gives the patient the characteristic "Popeye" appearance (enlarged forearms reminiscent of the cartoon character Popeye).

A facioscapulohumeral distribution of weakness may be seen in a number of neuromuscular disorders, and careful investigation is necessary to establish a correct diagnosis. Van Winjngaarden and Bethlem (1971) in a study of 17 cases of FSH syndrome found that seven were due to dystrophy, five to myotubular myopathy, two to myasthenia gravis, one to rod disease, one to central core disease and one to mitochondrial myopathy. Some spinal muscular atrophies may also have an "FSH distribution". Needless to say, all cases of FSH syndrome should have a muscle biopsy and electrodiagnostic evaluation.

The lower limbs are ultimately affected with an average of 10 to 15 years elapsing from the time of onset until such involvement occurs. In most cases, the dystrophic process descends from the shoulder girdle, skipping over the hip musculature to produce distal lower extremity weakness (Kazakov et al, 1974). Foot drop and steppage gait develop as a result of weakness of the peroneal and tibialis anterior muscles. This variety is sometimes referred to as facioscapuloperoneal dystrophy. Less commonly, the hip girdle musculature bears the brunt of the descending dystrophy. In such instances, the distal musculature is generally spared. The disease rarely involves cardiac or smooth muscle.

Because the disorder is usually slowly progressive, most patients lead productive lives, adapting themselves to their disability. However, there is a second form of FSH dystrophy which differs considerably from the classic variety just described. In some individuals, the disease is noted from early infancy. Facial weakness, with inability to close the eyes or suck properly, is the first indication that something is wrong. Frequently these patients are misdiagnosed as Möbius syndrome. However, with the development of girdle weakness, the correct diagnosis becomes more obvious. Such individuals are commonly confined to a wheelchair by age 10 years.

Laboratory Studies

Serum muscle enzymes

Approximately 50 percent of patients with FSH dystrophy wil have elevation of their serum CPK. Creatine phosphokinase elevations when they occur are two to four times above the normal range (Munsat et al, 1972).

Electrodiagnostic tests

Needle electromyographic study of involved muscle frequently shows a motor unit pattern of brief, small, abundant, polyphasic potentials (BSAPPs). Fibrillations may or may not be present. Nerve conduction velocities, as expected, are normal.

Muscle biopsy

Biopsy should be done in all cases of FSH syndrome to confirm the diagnosis and to exclude other than treatable disorders. The typical changes seen are nonspecific for FSH dystrophy but are similar to the other dystrophies. These changes include fiber size variablity, and moth-eaten and whorled fibers. It is of interest that in some patients there is a significant inflammatory reaction within the muscle similar to that seen in polymyositis (Munsat et al, 1972). In addition, esterase staining angulated fibers suggesting denervation are also occasionally encountered.

Treatment

Patients with FSH dystrophy whose biopsy demonstrates significant inflammatory changes probably deserve a trial of oral steroids. Some have had modest improvement with such therapy (Munsat et al, 1972). In general, however, the disease is relentlessly progressive.

Patients may benefit from surgical fixation of the scapulae which allows greater abduction of the arms. In addition, braces for foot drop may further aid the patient in his daily activities. Physiotherapy is helpful in preventing contractures and in maintaining strength in the muscles not affected.

LIMB GIRDLE DYSTROPHY

The term "limb girdle dystrophy" includes a heterogeneous group of disorders linked only by their common distribution of weakness and similar histologic changes in their muscle. Otherwise, the variability in age of onset, rate of progression, severity, and mode of transmission is so great that it is doubtful that they represent a single nosological entity.

The limb girdle syndrome may have its onset anytime from the second to beyond the fourth decade. Weakness usually begins in the pelvo-femoral muscles and after a variable period of time, involves the shoulder girdle. The "syndrome" varies in its degree of severity from family to family.

Muscle histology in this group of disorders is characterized by variability in fiber size, fiber splitting, profuse internal nuclei, and moth-eaten and whorled fibers. A variable inflammatory response with moderate number of necrotic fibers is also commonly seen (Brooke, 1973).

CONGENITAL MUSCULAR DYSTROPHY

The nosologic status of congenital muscular dystrophy (CMD) has been controversial. However, the consistent clinical and pathological features of these patients probably justify the consideration of CMD as a specific entity.

The disease probably has its most active and progressive phase in the fetus prior to birth. Diminished fetal movements in the last trimester of pregnancy are common. The infant with CMD is hypotonic, with generalized muscle weakness and multiple joint contractures (arthrogryposis). There is no calf hypertrophy and cranial musculature is generally spared except for mild facial weakness. Motor development is delayed, but most children with the disease improve in strength with maturity. Language and intellectual milestones are achieved on schedule. The disorder is believed to be familial following an autosomal recessive pattern of inheritance.

Laboratory studies are indicated in all such infants in order to exclude other more treated causes of "the floppy infant syndrome" (see Figure 5-1). Serum creatine phosphokinase levels are generally elevated while electro diagnostic tests and muscle pathology are supportive of a primary myopathic process.

DISTAL MYOPATHY

This is an uncommon familial disorder (autosomal dominant) characterized by slowly progressive *distal* muscle weakness. The disease usually has its onset in the third or fourth decade of life. Initially, symptoms are noted in either the

Table 4-1. Myopathies with Prominent Distal Limb Involvement

myotonic atrophy
type I fiber hypotrophy with central nuclei
rod disease
scapuloperoneal variety of facioscapulohumeral
  dystrophy
distal myopathy (dystrophy)

upper or lower limbs. Involvement of the distal upper extremities produces difficulty manipulating small objects (i.e., keys and buttoms). Distal lower limb disease results in a foot drop, an abnormal gait, and difficulty in rising on the toes. Proximal musculature may become mildly affected later in the course of the illness.

Cranial muscles are invariably spared. The disease is slowly progressive but never incapacitating. It neither shortens the lifespan nor the useful working life of the patient.

Because of the prominent distal weakness, cases may be confused with motor neuron disease (i.e., amyotrophic lateral sclerosis), familial neuropathies (i.e., Charcot-Marie-Tooth disease), acquired motor neuropathies (i.e., lead neuropathy), and other myopathies with distal manifestations (see Table 4-1). Laboratory studies are helpful in excluding these entities. Electrodiagnostic studies on patients with distal myopathy typically reveal normal conduction velocities and short duration polyphasic voluntary potentials (BSAPPs). Myotonic discharges, fasciculations and fibrillations are not found, and their absence exclude myotonic atrophy and motor neuron disease. The normal nerve conduction velocities and absence of giant potentials make the diagnosis of Charcot-Marie-Tooth disease unlikely. The remaining myopathies can be differentiated clinically (i.e., patients with type I fiber hypotrophy with central nuclei and rod disease usually have bony abnormalities) and by muscle biopsy. In the muscle tissue of patients with distal myopathy, one seem rimmed vacuoles which appear in the center of numerous fibers (Kumamoto et al, 1983). These are similar to the vacuoles seen in oculopharyngeal dystrophy. In addition, the muscle tissue shows all the changes associated with the dystrophies (i.e., fiber size variability, increased number of fibers with internal nuclei, fiber splitting and necrosis, and increased endomysial connective tissue). Neurogenic features (i.e., angulated fibers and fiber type grouping) are not found and this is further evidence against motor neuron disease and chronic axonal neuropathies.

CHAPTER 5

Morphologically Distinct "Myopathies" and Malignant Hyperthermia

TYPE I FIBER HYPOTROPHY WITH CENTRAL NUCLEI

Several groups of investigators have described a clinically heterogenous neuromuscular disease characterized histologically by small type I fibers and abundant internal nuclei. Spiro et al (1966) used the term "myotubular myopathy" for the disorder in the belief that the main pathology consisted of fibers resembling fetal myotubes. Sher et al (1967) reported their cases under the title "centronuclear myopathy" because they considered the presence of many centrally placed nuclei as the most characteristic feature. Engel et al (1968) argued against both these names. "Myotubular myopathy" they felt was not acceptable because there are important differences between true myotubes and the changes seen in the disease. The term centronuclear myopathy was equally inappropriate because many neuromuscular diseases are characterized by fibers with internal nuclei. Instead, they preferred calling the disorder "type I fiber hypotrophy with central nuclei" (IHCN). Although cumbersome, this latter term is more precise and avoids use of the word "myopathy" which implies a primary disorder of muscle. That the word myopathy be omitted from the title is advantageous because it is now believed that the disorder is secondary to defective neurotrophic influences on maturing muscle fibers.

Clinical Presentation: Signs and Symptoms

The patients with IHCN reported to date are clinically heterogenous. Such pleomorphic manifestations imply that IHCN is either an entity with a wide clinical expression or a syndrome consisting of more than one disease. Serratrice et al (1978) proposed a classification of IHCN according to age of onset and clinical characteristics. They postulated three forms:

1. an early type presenting at birth with hypotonia, diffuse weakness, and areflexia,
2. a more common variety beginning in early childhood,
3. a late type with onset in the third decade and a benign course.

With the infantile variety, the afflicted baby is floppy, feeds poorly, and is noted to have generalized weakness. There is usually significant cardiopulmonary involvement which leads to death between the ages of two days and 18 months. Most of these cases are inherited in an x-linked recessive pattern or are sporadic. Decreased fetal movements and polyhydramnios are frequent forerunners to the birth of such a child. The early childhood form, the most common type, generally appears after age two years. There is weakness of proximal and distal limb muscles as well as of cranial nerve musculature. Facial diplegia, ptosis, and impaired extraocular movements are prominent features. Disease progression is slow.

The late-onset variety is the most benign of the three. Such patients generally exhibit proximal and distal limb weakness (sometimes with greater involvement distally) without impairment of cranial structures. The illness tends to have a slowly progressive course. Most cases are familial (autosomal dominant). Other manifestations that may be seen in IHCN include calf pseudohypertrophy, myotonia, seizures, and/or dysmorphic features.

Laboratory Studies

The infantile variety of IHCN is one of the many disorders in the differential diagnosis of the floppy baby (see Figure 5-1). Muscle biopsy and electrodiagnostic studies are mandatory in order to exclude other more treatable causes of congenital hypotonia.

Electromyography

Electrodiagnostic studies in patients with IHCN most commonly shows a pattern of *b*rief, *s*mall, *a*bundant, *p*olyphaisc *p*otentials (BSAPPs). In addition, spontaneous fibrillations may be recorded in resting muscle.

Muscle biopsy

In IHCN, the histologic pattern of the muscle tissue defines the disease. Typically one observes abundant small fibers with internal nuclei. By histochemical staining, it is found that fiber types are less distinct than expected, but nearly all the type I fibers are small while the type II fibers are of normal size. In addition, type I fiber predominance (or type II paucity) is usually found (see Figure 5-2).

Carriers of the disease may have histologic abnormalities in their muscle

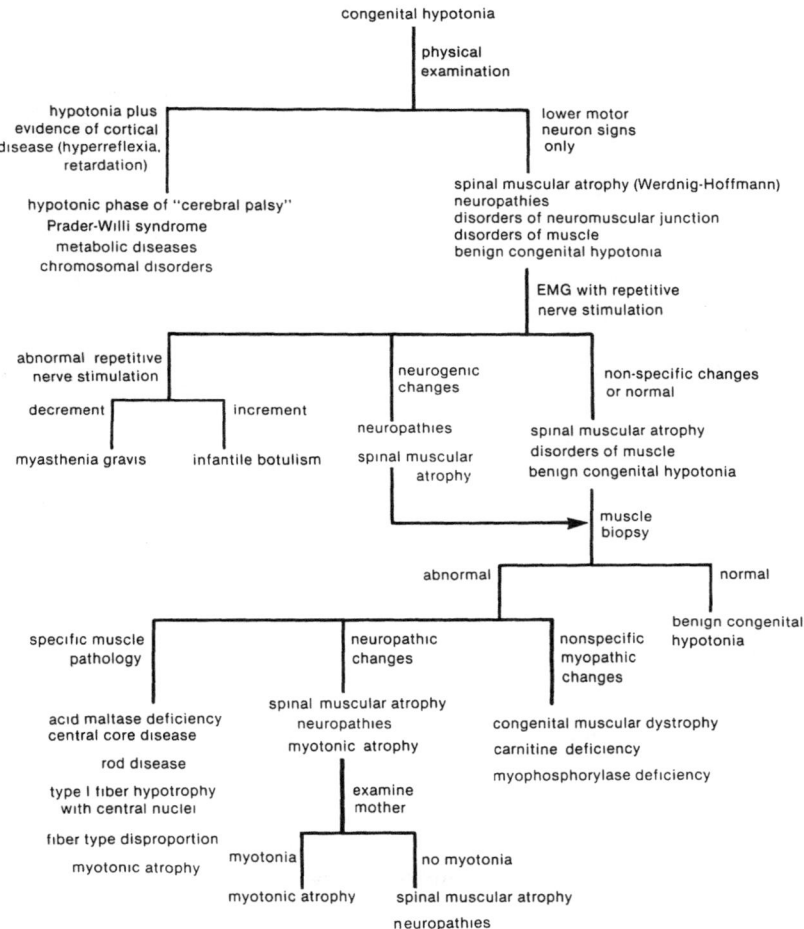

Figure 5-1. Summary flow chart. Symptom: congenital hypotonia (the floppy infant).

tissue including numerous small round type I fibers with or without central nuclei (Barth et al, 1975).

Serum muscle enzymes

Muscle enzymes are usually normal in IHCN although the CPK may be mildly elevated in some cases.

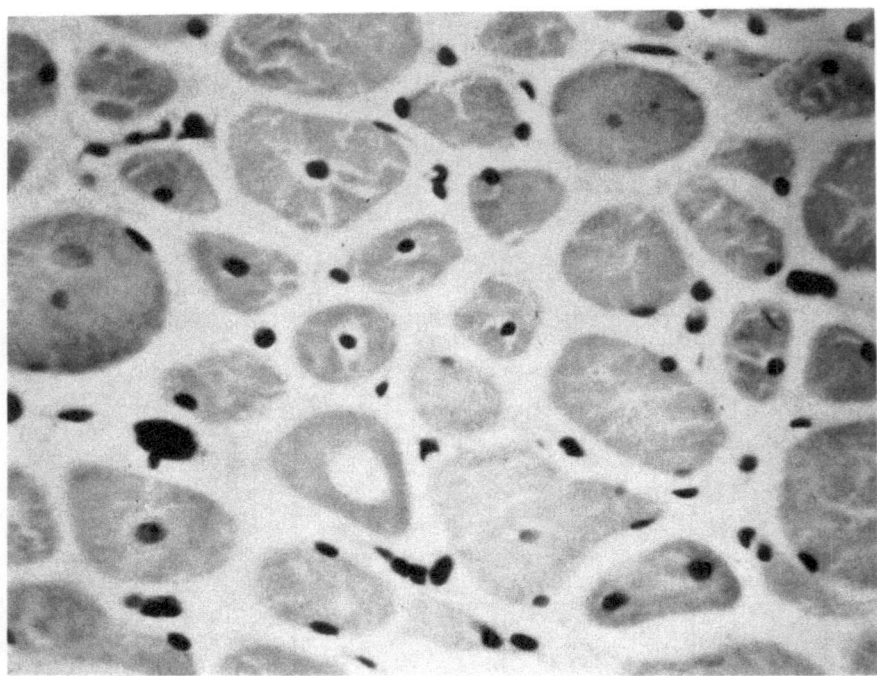

Figure 5-2. Muscle biopsy—type I fiber hypotrophy with central nuclei. Note the abundant small rounded fibers and numerous fibers with internal nuclei.

Pathophysiology

In normal embryonic development, muscle fibers form by fusion of mononucleated myoblasts to make a multinucleated myotube. The myotube is of small diameter, and in cross section, contains a thin peripheral rim of myofibrils surrounding a central axis of nuclei and intermyofibrillar components (mitochondria and reticulum). With further development, the myofibrils gradually fill the entire diameter and the nuclei migrate peripherally to occupy a subsarcolemmal position. All these stages can occur in non-innervated muscle fibers. Normally the myotube becomes innervated at 14 to 24 weeks of gestation, and it is the influence of the lower motor neuron that determines which fiber type (I or II) the myotube will develop into. By 28 weeks the fibers have enlarged, and can be differentiated histochemically into two approximately equal groups (types I and II). Thus, muscle fiber maturation is dependent on innervation.

It is postulated that in IHCN there is a subtle defect of neuronal influences upon which maturation of type I fibers is more dependent. It is suggested that the type I lower motor neurons innervate the hypotrophic fibers and transform them histochemically to type I fibers (a proof they are not myotubes), but these motor neurons are not able to promote peripheralization of the nuclei and growth to the normal diameter. Hence the hypothetical defect is attributed mainly to impairment of the trophic maturing influence of type I motor neurons.

In favor of this neurogenic hypothesis are the following:

1. an animal model of the disease produced by denervating muscle in newborn rats (Engel and Karpati, 1968),

2. the presence of EMG changes of denervation (i.e., fibrillations),

3. the lack of usual features of myopathy (muscle fiber necrosis and regeneration, endomysial connective tissue proliferation, and elevated CPK values).

A more detailed discussion on the pathogenesis of IHCN is provided by Engel (1977).

Treatment

Until recently there was no treatment for this disorder. However, Askanas et al (1979) discovered that muscle tissue from patients with IHCN had low levels of the enzyme adenylate cyclase. This enzyme converts ATP to cyclic AMP (see Figure 5-3), the latter compound serving as an important "second messenger" for a number of cellular functions including cell growth and differentiation. Since it is believed that there is neurotrophic regulation of cyclic nucleotide metabolism in muscle (Carlson, 1975), this biochemical abnormality would fit with the proposed neurogenic pathogenesis of the disease. Askanas et al postulated that patients with the disease might improve by increasing their cAMP levels and recommended administration of phthalazinol, a phosphodiesterase inhibitor. To date, two such infants have been treated with phthalazinol (70 mg./kg./day) and both have shown considerable improvement (Engel and Galdi, unpublished observation).

CENTRAL CORE DISEASE

In 1956, Shy and Magee described a family with an autosomal dominantly inherited non-progressive myopathy. The striking feature of the disease was the presence of non-staining "cores" in the muscle fibers. Hence, they called the disorder "central core disease" (CCD). Additional families with the disorder

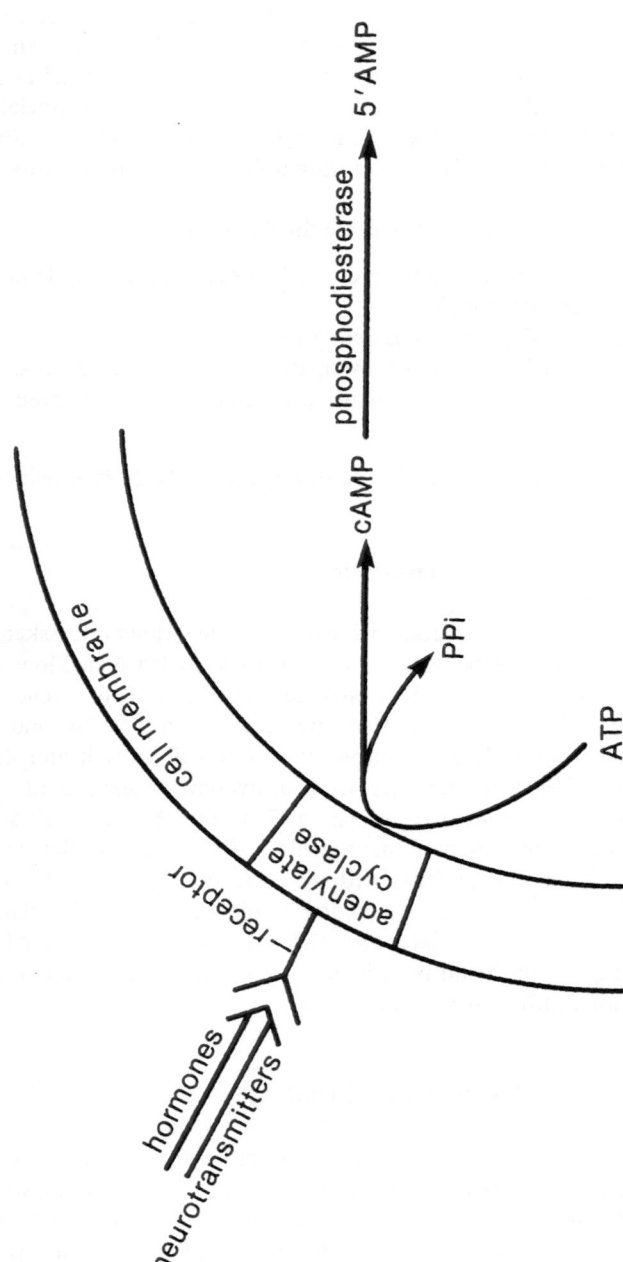

Figure 5-3. Synthesis and degradation of cyclic AMP. Cyclic AMP is formed from ATP by the action of adenylate cyclase. This enzyme is associated with the cell membrane and becomes activated when various hormones and/or neurotransmitters interact with the appropriate cell surface receptor. Cyclic AMP translates extracellular messages into intracellular responses. Its action is terminated by the enzyme phosphodiesterase.

have subsequently been described and it has become evident that central core disease has a variable clinical picture and may be in some cases, a clinically silent morphologic abnormality (Patterson et al, 1979). Furthermore, it appears that patients with the disorder are at risk of developing anesthetic-induced malignant hyperthermia.

Clinical Presentation: Signs and Symptoms

Central core disease may present in infancy with hypotonia and delayed motor milestones. Patients gradually acquire all the normal motor skills but remain mildly to moderately weak. This weakness is usually more prominent in the proximal limb musculature especially that of the lower extremities. Occasionally there is weakness of the facial musculature, but ocular, cardiac, and smooth muscles are not affected. Congenital hip dislocation, kyphoscoliosis, pes cavus, and recurrent patellar dislocations commonly occur in association with the disorder. The children remain slender and ofter short-statured, and they can seldom run or jump with any facility. Occasionally central core disease does not become clinically apparent until late adult life (Telerman-Toppet et al, 1973). In such instances, initial symptoms may be distal lower extremity weakness. In general, central core disease is not progressive and does not shorten lifespan.

In 1973, Denborough et al reported a case of central core disease in a 71-year-old patient whose family had ten members who had died from malignant hyperthermia. It soon became apparent that patients with CCD fall into a high risk category for malignant hyperthermia (Eng et al, 1978; Frank et al, 1980).

Malignant hyperthermia is an anesthetic-induced syndrome in which there is an explosive rise in body temperature, muscle rigidity, and necrosis. It can be provoked by the administration of skeletal muscle relaxants or inhalation anesthetics. Shortly after the triggering agent is administered, there is an extraordinary rise in body temperature, intense muscle rigidity, and metabolic acidosis. Complications include consumptive coagulopathy, renal failure (secondary to muscle necrosis and myoglobinuria), and cardiac dysrhythmias. The mortality rate may be as high as 70 percent. Most patients with malignant hyperthermia do not have CCD and not all CCD patients experience malignant hyperthermia. However, all CCD patients and their relatives should be considered at risk and should undergo appropriate testing (i.e., muscle biopsy). Potential malignant hyperthermia patients who require surgery should have local or regional block, if possible. Lidocaine is not to be used but procaine is safe. If general anesthesia is necessary, halothane and/or succinycholine are to be avoided. Pre-treatment with dantrolene prior to the planned surgery is also recommended.

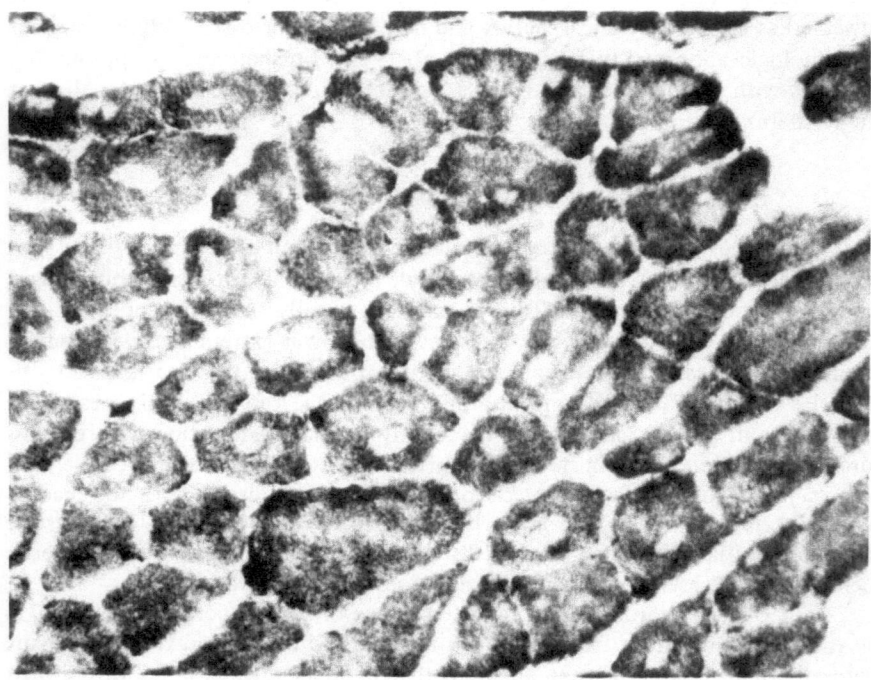

Figure 5-4. Muscle biopsy—central core disease (NADH-TR stain). Note the non-staining core regions in numerous fibers.

Laboratory Studies

Muscle biopsy

The characteristic finding in CCD is the abnormal core region in many fibers. The number of fibers with cores varies from a few to almost 100 percent in some instances. Cores occur only in type I fibers and may be eccentric in position or multiple in number.

Histochemically, the core region is unstained by reactions for mitochondrial oxidative enzymes (NADH-TR stain) and phosphorylase. (See Figure 5-4.)

In addition, there is usually an abnormally large percentage of type I fibers and a moderate number of small angulated fibers.

Electromyography

A pattern of *b*rief, *s*mall, *a*bundant, *p*olyphasic *p*otentials frequently is seen in patients with CCD (BSAPPs).

Serum muscle enzymes

Creatine phosphokinase levels are normal or mildly elevated in patients with CCD. The use of CPK levels to screen for patients with clinically silent CCD (yet at risk for malignant hyperthermia) is not reliable.

Pathophysiology

Currently it is believed that CCD represents an unusual type of "neuropathy" rather than a primary myopathy. It is postulated that the structural defect in the muscle is secondary to defective neural influences during embryonic differentiation of muscle fibers. In support of a neurogenic process are the observations that cores resemble target fibers (which are known to occur with neurogenic disease) and the fact that core/targetoid fibers have been demonstrated in cat soleus muscle three to five weeks after total denervation (Engel et al, 1966). In addition, the type I fiber predominance and the presence of small angulated fibers support a neurogenic process.

Treatment

There is no specific treatment of CCD. However, it is of the utmost importance to screen asymptomatic family members of patients with CCD and to identify those at risk for malignant hyperthermia. This may be best accomplished by muscle biopsy and in vitro exposure of excised muscle strips to halothane, caffeine, and/or suxmethonium (Ellis et al, 1972). Assay of myophosphorylase A levels in the muscle tissue (Willner et al, 1980) may also identify those at risk. Once these individuals have been identified, they should be instructed to wear medical alert bracelets attesting to the fact that they are subject to malignant hyperpyrexia.

ROD (NEMALINE) DISEASE

In 1963, Shy et al reported an infant who was floppy at birth and whose muscle fibers contained peculiar thread-like structures. Hence, they called the disease "nemaline myopathy" after the Greek word for thread (nema). Two variants of nemaline myopathy, or rod disease, are now recognized. In the congenital form, patients present at birth with hypotonia and proximal weakness that in most cases is not progressive. The more recently described adult-onset variety is characterized by the insidious development of weakness principally in a scapuloperoneal distribution (Feigenbaum and Munsat, 1970).

Rod disease appears to be inherited in either an autosomal dominant or autosomal recessive pattern. These two genetic varieties are indistinguishable

on a clinical or histopathologic basis. In addition, sporadic cases of the disease
do occur.

Clinical Presentation: Signs and Symptoms

Most commonly, the patient with rod disease presents at birth as a floppy
infant. In addition ot hypotonia and diffuse trunk and limb weakness (more
pronounced proximally) there may be respiratory difficulty and problems
with sucking and swallowing. Extraocular movements are generally well-pre-
served and there is no ptosis or sensory abnormality. Tendon reflexes are usually depressed or absent. Mentation is normal and helps to differentiate these
children from those with cerebral causes of hypotonia. In addition, bony deformities such as pes cavus and kyphoscoliosis may accompany the disorder.
Over 70 percent of affected children have a high arched palate.

As the child grows older, there is delayed achievement of motor milestones. However, in most cases, the weakness is not progressive or progresses
very slowly. Affected children tend to be of slender body habitus with long,
thin faces and dental malocclusion.

As previously mentioned, rod disease may have its onset in adolescence
or late adult life (Engel and Resnick, 1966; Brownell et al, 1978). In these
patients weakness usually begins in the muscles of the anterior tibial compart-
ment and shoulder girdle. Foot drop may be the earliest manifestation. Gradually the weakness becomes diffuse and generalized with preservation of the
bulbar musculature. The rate of disease progression in adult-onset form varies.
All reported cases are non-familial.

Laboratory Studies

Muscle biopsy

Muscle biopsy is paramount in arriving at the diagnosis. Most patients with
rod disease show type I fiber predominance. However, the most striking feature
is the presence of rod bodies in the center and periphery of numerous fibers (see
Figure 5-5). The number of fibers containing such rods varies from case to case
and from muscle to muscle in the same patient. The modified trichrome stain
of Engel and Cunningham stains these structures bright red.

Ultrastructurally, rods appear to be derived from the Z bands of sarcomeres.
Their exact chemical composition is unknown, but the major component may be
α-actinin (Schollmeyer et al, 1973).

It must be emphasized that rod bodies are not disease-specific but can be
found in a variety of neuromuscular (Afifi et al, 1965) and non-neuromuscular
disorders. What make them specific of rod disease is their great abundance and
the absence of other pathological changes.

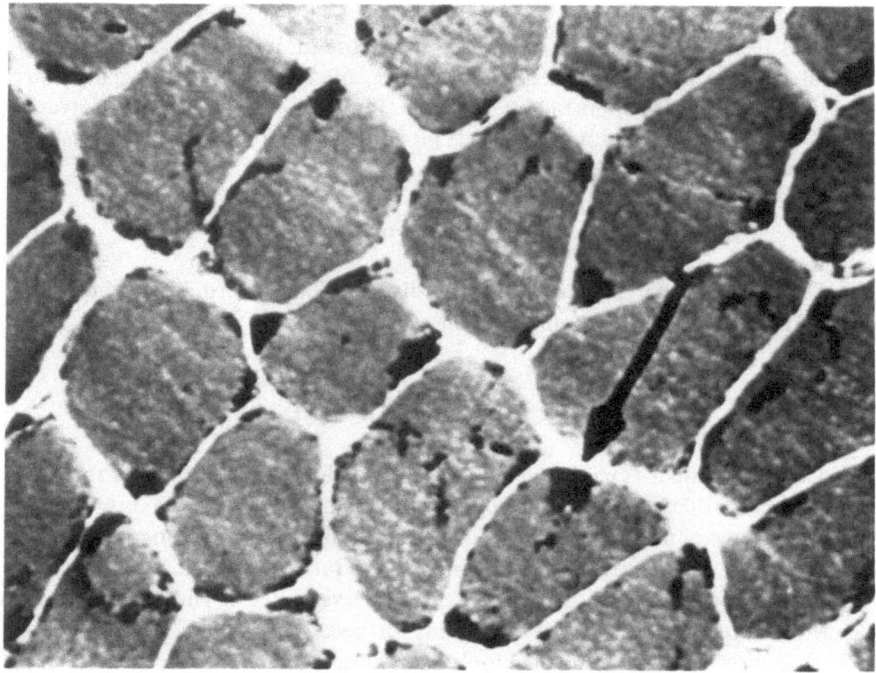

Figure 5-5. Muscle biopsy—rod disease (modified Gomon trichrome stain). Note the darkly staining rods in many fibers.

Electrodiagnostic studies

Patients with rod disease may have EMG evidence of denervation. Fibrillations, giant potentials, and incomplete interference patterns of maximum voluntary effort may be seen (Brownell et al, 1978). In other instances, a pattern of brief, small, overly abundant, polyphasic motor unit action potentials (BSAPPs) is evident. As expected, nerve conduction velocities are normal.

Serum muscle enzymes

Serum muscle enzyme concentrations are usually normal in cases of rod disease. Occasionally slight elevations of the serum CPK and aldolase has been noted.

Pathophysiology

It is believed that rod disease like central core disease and several other congenital "myopathies" is the result of a neurogenic rather than a myopathic process. This concept is supported by the EMG. Findings of denervation-renervation in many of the patients and of the type I fiber predominance are observed in their muscle biopsies.

Treatment

There is no specific treatment of rod disease. Corticosteroids have been tried in several patients, but without success.

CONGENITAL FIBER TYPE DISPROPORTION

Congenital fiber type disproportion is probably a syndrome rather than a disease. Most patients are born floppy with generalized muscle weakness and hypotonia. Bony abnormalities including congenital hip dislocations, kyphoscoliosis, and foot deformities are common, as are contractures. The weakness tends to be non-progressive or slowly progressive for several years. The disease is familial with either an autosomal dominant or recessive pattern of inheritance.

Diagnosis can be confirmed only by muscle biopsy. Typically one finds small type I fibers which are in disproprotionally greater numbers than the type II fibers.

MALIGNANT HYPERTHERMIA

Malignant hyperthermia (MH) is a syndrome in which there is an explosive rise in body temperature, severe muscle rigidity, and acidosis. In susceptible individuals it may be provoked by muscle relaxants (especially succinylcholine) and/or inhalation anesthetics (especially halothane). Strenuous physical activity may also induce attacks. The propensity to develop MH is inherited, usually in an autosomal dominant fashion. However, families with autosomal recessive patterns of inheritance as well as with sporadic cases have been observed. Some myopathies, including Duchenne's muscular dystrophy, the myotonias, and central core disease impart a risk of MH that is greater than the risk of the population at large. Study of an animal model of MH (porcine stress syndrome) has been helpful in elucidating the pathophysiology of the disorder.

Presently, the metabolic defect in MH is felt to lie in the sarcoplasmic reticulum which releases excess Ca^{++} and fails to reaccumulate Ca^{++} when exposed to certain exogenous agents. This results in generalized muscle rigidity and failure of relaxation, and available ATP is rapidly expended. The high concentration of sarcoplasmic Ca^{++} also appears to uncouple mitochondria resulting in excessive heat production without ATP regeneration.Because an episode of MH may be fatal, it is important to recognize its early clinical manifestations so that treatment can be promptly instituted. Equally important is the identification of those at risk so that appropriate precautions can be taken.

Clinical Presentation: Signs and Symptoms

Malignant hyperthermia usually occurs during elective surgery, e.g., orthopedic, dental, or other musculoskeletal procedures. It has been estimated to occur in from 1 in 15,000 to 1 in 50,000 patients who have been subjected to anesthesia (Gallant and Ahern, 1983). It may be triggered by an potent volatile anesthetic agent but onset is usually more abrupt when succinylcholine is also used. The earliest sign may be rigidity of the masseter muscles which inhibits easy tracheal intubation. Shortly thereafter, there is an extraordinary rise in body temperature (as high as 108°F), tachycardia, tachypnea, general muscle rigidity, and fasciculations. Intense muscle necrosis follows which leads to a marked increase in serum creatine phosphokinase, myoglobin, calcium, and potassium. A profound metabolic acidosis further complicates the picture. If appropriate treatment is not instituted, death is almost a certainty. Those who succumb have generally developed lethal cardiac dysrhythmias, renal failure, disseminated intravascular coagulation, and/or hypoxic-ischemic cerebral lesions.

The cornerstone of treatment of MH is its early recognition. An unexplained 1°C rise in body temperature in two successive 15 minute intervals is an ominous sign. The anesthesia and operation should be terminated immediately. Initial treatment is aimed at bringing down the body temperature and correcting the acidosis and hyperkalemia. A cooling blanket may suffice; however, if the temperature is very high, surface cooling with ice, rectal, and esophageal ice water lavage may be needed. The use of bicarbonate to control the acidosis and glucose/insulin infusions to correct the hyperkalemia are essential. Urinary output should be measured and diuresis maintained using volume loading or diuretics. Dantrolene is the only known specific therapeutic drug but it must be administered while there is still adequate muscle perfusion. Dantrolene attenuates Ca^{++} release without interfering with its re-uptake. It appears to act on the transverse tubules and sarcoplasmic reticulum. For MH the recommended dose is 1-2 mg/kg intravenously every 15 minutes to a total dose of 10 mg/kg. Since the drug has a short half-life (approximately five hours) it should be continued for from 12 to 24 hours after the control of MH.

Screening for Susceptibility

Most MH-affected people appear normal and have no overt evidence of neuromuscular disease. However, it appears that patients with Duchenne's muscular dystrophy, myotonia, central core disease, and Burkitt's lymphoma are at increased risk. Such individuals and those with a family history of MH should be screened. Serum creatine phosphokinase levels are inadequate for this purpose. Muscle biopsy is the only way to determine susceptibility. The excised muscle tissue is exposed in a temperature controlled bath to halothane, caffeine, and halothane/caffeine. These agents promote Ca^{++} release from the sarcoplasmic reticulum. Muscle tissue from patients prone to MH will develop contractures at much lower concentrations of these agents than will normal muscle.

Those at risk who require surgery should be pretreated with dantrolene 4-7 mg/kg/day given in divided doses and started at least 24 hours pre-operatively. The safe anesthetics include nitrous oxide, thiopental, and other barbiturates, opiates, and pancuronium. Potent volatile agents, depolarizing relaxants, and ketamine should be avoided. Excellent reviews of the malignant hyperpyrexia syndrome are provided by Gronert (1980) and Nelson and Flewellen (1983).

CHAPTER 6

Myotonia and Myotonic Disorders

MYOTONIA

Clinical Characteristics

Myotonia is the delayed relaxation of muscles following voluntary contraction (action myotonia) or mechanical stimulation (percussion myotonia). Action myotonia can be demonstrated by asking the patient to release a tightly clinched fist quickly or by having a patient look down after sustained upgaze. (The upper lids will remain hung for up to 10 seconds.) Typically, action myotonia improves with repeated activity although an occasional patient will report the reverse situation (paradoxical myotonia). Exposure to cold frequently worsens the problem while heat has the opposite effect. Percussion myotonia is useful diagnostically when elicited by the examiner but does not cause symptoms. It can be evoked in the thenar eminences, tongue, and wrist extensors by briskly tapping these areas with a reflex hammer. A positive response is seen as sustained dimpling in the region struck with the hammer. Action and percussion myotonia are not equally expressed in myotonic patients and a specific search for each type is necessary on routine physical examination.

Patients with symptomatic myotonia generally complain of muscle stiffness and slowness of movement. This may be severe enough to seriously restrict physical activity.

There are a number of diseases associated with myotonia, including (1) myotonic atrophy (dystrophy), (2) myotonia congenita, (3) paramyotonia congenita, (4) hyperkalemic periodic paralysis (see Chapter 7), and (5) Schwartz-Jampel syndrome. Additionally, myotonia may be produced by drugs (i.e., clofibrate), and may appear as a remote effect of lung carcinoma or as secondary to thyroid dysfunction (Venables et al, 1978).

Electrical Characteristics

The myotonic response has several electrical properties which make it readily identifiable with EMG studies. Characteristic properties are spontaneous high frequency repetitive discharges that show a recurrent variation in amplitude and frequency. The waxing and waning in amplitude and frequency are responsible for the associated dive-bomber-like sound heard over the EMG loudspeaker. The myotonic response may appear spontaneously or be evoked by voluntary movement, percussion, needle movement, electrical stimulation, or cold (Goodgold and Eberstein, 1977). Bizarre high frequency discharges without variation in amplitude or frequency are called pseudomyotonia and are seen with chronic denervation.

Pathophysiology

Myotonia is of muscular origin and does not depend on motor nerve activity as indicated by its presence following curarization. It is believed to result from an unstable sarcolemmal membrane which is abnormally sensitive to discharge, by a variety of electrical, chemical, and mechanical stimuli. Experimental observations have clearly implicated a marked reduction in sarcolemmal chloride conductance as a causal factor in a group of myotonic syndromes including human myotonia congenita, hereditary goat myotonia, and myotonia produced by aromatic carboxylic acid (Barchi, 1975). This defect in chloride conductance has not been found in human myotonic atrophy or paramyotonia congenita. The diminished conductance to Cl^- hinders effective membrane repolarization because the preceding depolarizing effect of increased Na^+ conductance can only be counterbalanced by an enhanced K^+ conductance. The membrane is thus deprived of the normal increase Cl^- conductance that helps effect membrane repolarization and muscle relaxation. Experimental support of this theory is found in isolated muscle preps which are observed to undergo spontaneous repetitive activity when the Cl^- in the fluid bath is replaced with an impermeant anion (Falk and Landa, 1960). Theoretical considerations suggest that myotonia could be caused by primary abnormalities on the Na^+ conductance system. Recent work on paramyotonia congenita indicates that this disorder may be an example of such a defect. In this disease there may be a temperature-dependent abnormality in the sodium conductance pathway (Lehman-Horn et al, 1981).

In myotonic atrophy, abnormalities have been reported in the rate of Ca^{++} transport (Plishker et al, 1978) and the activities of the Na^+-K^+ ATPase (Niebroj-Dobosz, 1976). However, the precise pathophysiology remains an enigma.

A biochemical alteration in the muscle membrane may prove to be the underlying defect in the myotonic disorders. A genetically determined chemical change in the cholesterol component of the membrane is suggested by the fact that myotonia can be produced by agents that inhibit cholesterol synthesis (Winer et al, 1965). However, detailed biochemical analysis of myotonic muscle membrane still requires further elucidation.

MYOTONIC ATROPHY (STEINERT'S DISEASE)

Myotonic atrophy (MyA) is one of the more common myopathies and certainly the most frequent of the myotonias. Its prevalence rate is approximately 3.3 per 100,000. It is a multisystem disease involving not only skeletal muscle but myocardial and visceral smooth muscle as well. Furthermore, MyA affects bones, eyes, hair, metabolic and endocrine function. Abnormalities of intelligence and behavior complete its multifaceted picture.

The disease is transmitted as a monogenic autosomal dominant trait. Both sexes are affected with equal frequency. Because its gene expressivity varies and penetrance is not always complete, the clinical picture of the disease is variable. Relatives of patients with unequivocal MyA may have only minimal evidence of the disorder, with cataracts, facial weakness, hyporeflexia, and/or ECG abnormalities the only manifestations (Pryse-Phillips et al, 1982). Patients with these partial syndromes may not exhibit clinical or electrical myotonia.

The initial symptoms usually appear between the ages of 15 and 40, although a form of MyA may be present at birth (neonatal myotonic atrophy). Most patients die before the age of 60, usually from cardiorespiratory complications.

Clinical Presentation: Signs and Symptoms

Typically, the symptoms of MyA are not apparent until adolescence or early adult life. Patients may manifest evidence of myotonia early in the course of their disease. Failure of grasp relaxation when turning a doorknob or after a handshake may be bothersome but seldom incapacitating. Muscle stiffness and cramping are not significant problems and it is only when distal weakness and atrophy appear that the patient seeks medical attention.

Skeletal muscle involvement in MyA is highly selective. The facial, oropharyngeal, masticatory, and distal muscles of the upper and lower limbs are among the earliest and most severely involved. Foot extensor muscles are particularly weak with foot drop, an abnormal gait, and Achilles tendon contractures as common problems. The comparative preservation of strength and bulk in the proximal musculature is striking in the early stages of the disease.

Facial diplegia produces a flat sagging face and in association with the hollow temples and ptosis accounts for the sad "myopathic" facies. The mouth is frequently kept open and is shaped like an inverted "V" (shark mouth). Weak-

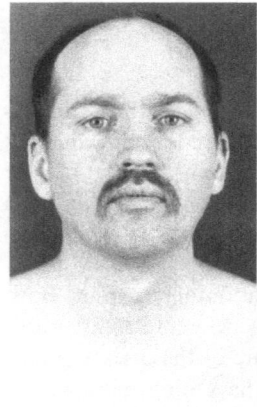 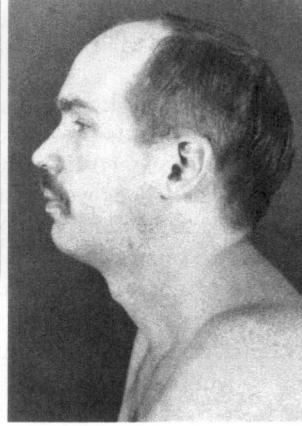

Figure 6-1. A patient with myotonic atrophy. Note the frontal balding, left ptosis, and wasting of the neck and distal limb musculature.

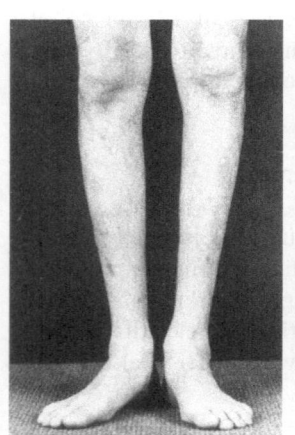 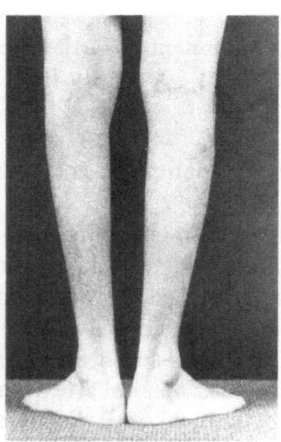 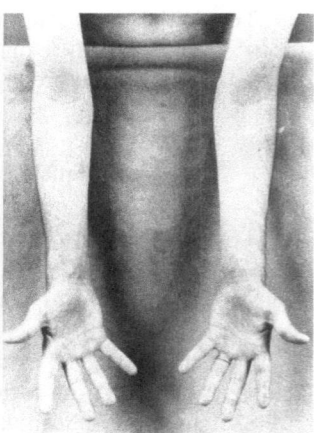

ness and atrophy of the sternocleidomastoids may be striking and they are often reduced to thin fibrous bands. With the passage of time, the oropharyngeal muscles become involved producing dysarthria, dysphagia, and nasal regurgitation (see Figure 6-1a).

Myotonia is not as marked as in myotonia congenita and is usually limited to the distal limb musculature and face. It rarely produces a grave handicap for the patient. However, myotonia of the diaphragm and intercostal muscles may compromise respiratory function. As the muscles become weaker and more atrophic, the myotonia disappears.

Myocardial involvement is frequent, occurring in approximately 60 percent of cases. Dysrhythmias and/or conduction abnormalities are commonly found, and more recently an association between MyA and mitral valve prolapse has been appreciated (Winters et al, 1976).

Other clinical manifestations of MyA are briefly discussed below and are more thoroughly reviewed in a paper by Zellweger and Jonasescu (1973).

Smooth muscle

The upper and lower GI tract as well as the urinary excretory pathways may be affected in the disease. Hypoperistalsis leads to dilatation of the esophagus and colon, and to constipation. Delayed relaxation of internal sphincters can produce urinary retention and gall bladder dysfunction with stone formation.

Eye

Cataracts usually appear between the ages of 25 and 40 and are found in over 90 percent of MyA patients. Such lenticular opacities are generally in the subcapsular part of the posterior pole.

Scalp and bone

Frontal baldness is frequently found in the adult with MyA. Radiological abnormalities of the skull include diffuse thickening of the cranial vault (hyperostosis cranii), localized thickening of the frontal bones (hyperostosis frontalis interna), large sinuses, and small sella turcica.

Endocrone and metabolic function

Hypogonadism is the foremost endocrine disorder. The male genitalia, especially the gonads, are small. Female MyA patients often have menstrual irregularities and both sexes are commonly infertile.

Abnormal glucose tolerance and elevated fasting levels of serum insulin are also encountered. Additionally, low plasma IgG concentrations may be noted (Engel, 1966).

Intelligence and behavior

The incidence of mental subnormality is high in MyA. Many patients have I.Q.'s in the 50 to 75 range. Deviant behavior is another feature of the disease and varies from indifference to hostile agressive behavior. Hypersomnia has also been reported in patients with MyA (Hansatia and Frens, 1981).

In most instances, the patient with MyA can be diagnosed as he walks into the physician's office. The premature frontal balding, sagging facies, ptotic lids, and temporalis/sternocleidomastoid atrophy give an unmistakable appearance to these patients. Occasionally, because of the pronounced distal weakness and wasting, the patient may be confused with cases of axonal neuropathies, motor neuron disease, rod myopathy, or distal myopathy (see Table 4-1). A careful physical examination will, in most cases, differentiate these entities. However, laboratory studies may be needed to confirm the diagnosis of MyA.

Laboratory Studies

Muscle biopsy

Muscle tissue of the adult MyA patient is characterized by small type I fibers and large type II fibers. Internal nuclei are frequent and are probably more numerous in MyA than in almost any other neuromuscular disease (Dubowitz and Brooke, 1973) (see Figure 6-2). Histologic changes that characterize the dystrophies (i.e., necrotic fibers, increased endomysial connective tissue, and "regen-degen" fibers) are not seen. The name myotonic atrophy (referring to the type I fiber atrophy) more accurately describes the pathology and therefore, is preferred to myotonic dystrophy.

Electromyography

Electromyographic studies reveal myotonic discharges which are present in many muscles but most exuberant in hand muscles. Such discharges are not found in axonal neuropathies, motor neuron disease, or other myopathies with distal weakness. With advanced disease, low amplitude, short duration polyphasic voluntary potentials become apparent (BSAPPs).

Serum muscle enzymes

Serum levels of CPK, aldolase and the transaminases (GOT and GPT) are normal in the majority of cases of MyA. Mild elevations of CPK are found in rare instances while very high levels speak against the diagnosis.

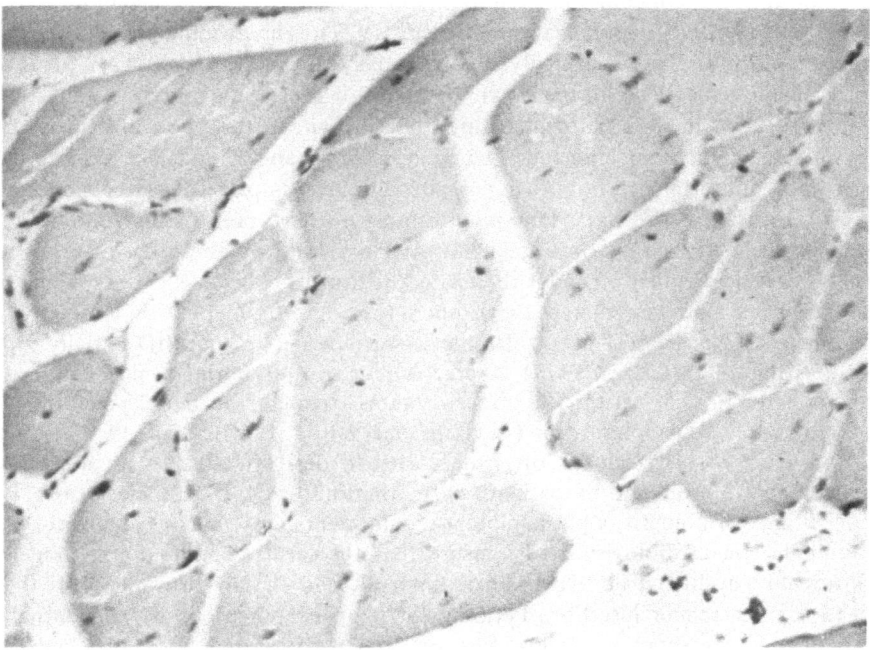

Figure 6-2. Muscle biopsy from a patient with MyA. Note the numerous fibers with internal nuclei.

Prognosis and Treatment

The prognosis is variable although the majority of patients are confined to a wheelchair 20 years after the onset of the disease. Life expectancy is shorter than for the general population at large because of life-threatening cardiorespiratory complications. (For summary, see Figure 6-3.)

Proper management of patients with MyA can be divided into two aspects:

1. treatment of the myotonia, the motor disability and medical complications, and

2. genetic counselling.

Effective therapy in MyA is limited by the fact that many patients are not significantly benefited by treatment of the myotonia since their motor weakness progresses. However, in the patient with symptomatic myotonia, relief can be obtained with a variety of drugs including phenytoin, procainamide and acetazolamide. Phenytoin produces its therapeutic effect probably by decreasing net

Na^+ influx during membrane excitation which makes the membrane more resistant to repetitive depolarization (Griggs, 1977). The recommended dose is between 200 and 400 mg. daily in two equally divided doses (Munsat, 1967). Procainamide has also been shown to stabilize muscle membranes and is an effective agent in the treatment of myotonia. However, its use is limited by its toxic side effects which include insomnia, anxiety, and a lupus-like syndrome. It is most important to note that procainamide may impair myocardial conduction. Thus it may be hazardous in patients who have pre-existing conduction defects as is commonly the case in MyA. Phenytoin, on the other hand, promotes cardiac conduction and is therefore, the drug of choice.

In some patients, therapy with phenytoin or procainamide is ineffective. In such cases, a trial of acetazolamide is warranted (125 mg BID initially, up to 250 mg TID) (Griggs, 1977). Acetazolamide, by promoting a mild kaluresis and a reduction in serum K^+ concentrations, renders the muscle membrane more resistant to depolarization (Leyburn and Walton, 1960).

A team of physicians is often necessary to deal effectively with the multiple medical problems of patients with myotonic atrophy. In most cases, a consulting cardiologist, ophthalmologist, endocrinologist, and psychiatrist are required. The cardiologist should insure that the cardiac conduction system is thoroughly evaluated at two to three intervals and should also advise on the need for pacemaker insertion. Periodic slit lamp examinations by an ophthalmologist are necessary to follow the progression of cataract formation and to determine when surgical intervention is appropriate. An endocrinologist with a special interest in insulin resistant diabetes mellitus is essential, because frequently patients with myotonic atrophy fail to respond to the standard diabetic treatment regimens. Because the illness is familial and patients know what lies ahead from memories of older affected relatives, a depressive psychosis commonly appears in the course of the disease. Psychotherapy and pharmacologic treatment of the mood disorder may be necessary.

Genetic counselling is an important part of the management of patients with MyA. Such individuals should be warned that there is an even chance of any child developing the disorder. Early detection of the disease before the onset of overt signs and symptoms is important, because many patients have children prior to the onset of symptoms and thus are deprived of proper counselling. Early suspect cases can often be unmasked by a careful physical examination, slit lamp evaluation in search of cataracts, and EMG studies (Polgar et al, 1972).

NEONATAL MYOTONIC ATROPHY (DYSTROPHY)

Myotonic atrophy (MyA) is generally considered to be a disease of adult life. However a congenital form of the illness has been recognized whose clinical features differ considerably from those seen in later life. The clinical picture of

HISTORY   30 y.o. male with difficulty relaxing hand grasp, weakness and wasting in hands and tripping when climbing up stairs. Family history positive for cataracts.

PHYSICAL

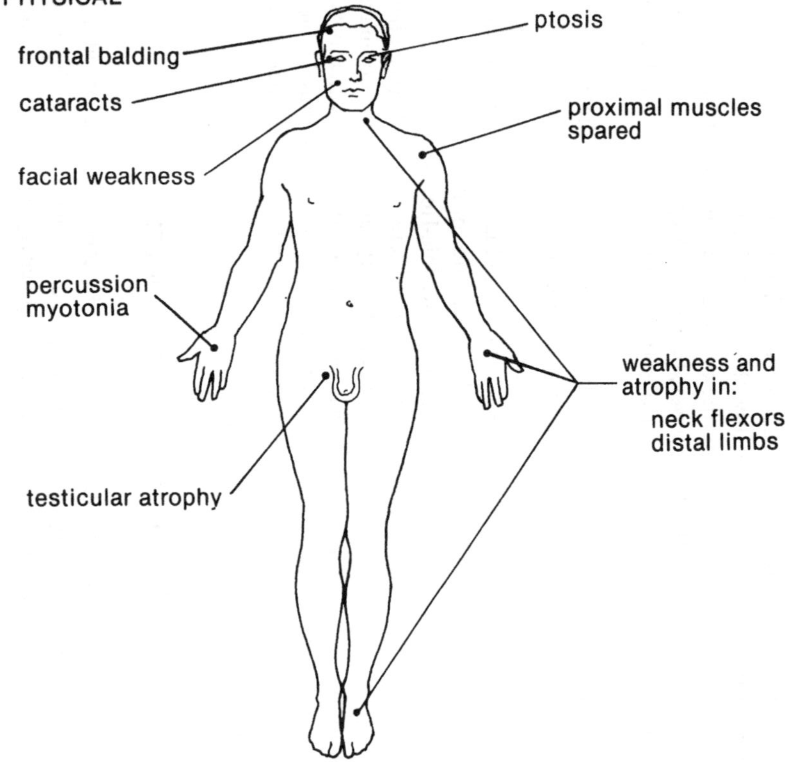

- ptosis
- frontal balding
- cataracts
- facial weakness
- percussion myotonia
- proximal muscles spared
- weakness and atrophy in: neck flexors, distal limbs
- testicular atrophy

LAB

Normal CPK, aldolase

EMG: myotonia with waxing and waning of the amplitude and frequency

Biopsy: type I fiber hypo-trophy with type II fiber hypertrophy, internal nuclei

Other: ECG with prolonged PR interval, abnormal skull X-rays

TREATMENT

phenytoin 200 - 400 mg daily

PROGNOSIS

slowly progressive disability wheelchair bound in 20 to 30 years after onset

Figure 6-3.   Summary of myotonic dystrophy (atrophy).

neonatal MyA is dominated by hopotonia rather than myotonia and may result in severe, even fatal, respiratory problems in the newborn.

It is of interest that in the majority of cases of congenital MyA the mother is found to be the affected parent. It has been hypothesized that the disease results from an intrauterine maternal factor acting upon the fetus carrying the gene for MyA (Harper and Dyken, 1972). Congenital abnormalities occur in a considerable proportion of such infants and there is an increased incidence of hydramnios complicating these pregnancies.

Clinical Presentation: Signs and Symptoms

The majority of patients with neonatal MyA present as floppy infants with delayed motor development. Difficulty with breathing and swallowing are noted from birth. Facial diplegia is common and seen in almost 90 percent of cases (Harper, 1975). Talipes and other congential malformations are also frequently a part of the syndrome. The absence of some of the cardinal features of the adult form of the disease, notably the myotonia, is important. These infants do not develop myotonia before the age of 1 year and only 10 to 20 percent do so by age 5 (Harper 1975). However, between the ages of 5 to 10 years. all develop myotonia. Cataracts are not observed in the early stages of the congenital variety.

Prognosis in these infants is unfavorable and many die in the neonatal period. Survivors show delayed motor development and approximately 70 percent are mentally retarded. Some patients, however, improve during the first decade of life but subsequently experience a gradual progression of their muscle weakness and wasting together with the appearance of myotonia.

The differential diagnosis includes Wednig-Hoffmann disease, various congential "myopathies", and the hypotonia of cerebral anoxia (see Figure 5-1). Even in the absence of a positive family history of MyA, the combination of hypotonia, facial diplegia, and such factors as talipes and hydramnios should allow a clinical diagnosis. Electromyographic studies and muscle biopsy are useful in excluding the other entities mentioned earlier as diagnostic possibilities.

MYOTONIA CONGENITA (THOMSEN'S DISEASE)

In 1876, Asmus Thomsen, a Danish physician, first described a peculiar disorder characterized by muscle camping and stiffness. He was able to describe the disease, which now bears his name, so precisely because he himself was afflicted.

Myotonia congenita (MC) is a rare disease with a prevalence rate between

0.3 and 0.6 per 100,000 people. Two varieties that differ in their modes of inheritance and clinical characteristics are now recognized. The autosomal dominant form as described by Thomsen has its onset early in life, while the more common autosomal recessive type first recognized by Becker in 1966 begins later and is characterized by more severe muscle impairment. Differentiating between the two forms is of practical significance for genetic counselling. In Thomsen's variety, one can predict that approximately one-half of the offspring will be affected, whereas if the disease is of the autosomal recessive type, the risk to future generations is negligible.

In both varieties of MC muscle stiffness is the predominant symptom from which the individual suffers. Patients complain of difficulty in walking and running, with frequent falls, and of stiffness and clumsiness particularly when attempting movements following prolonged periods of rest. Unlike those with myotonic atrophy, patients with MC do not develop significant weakness, multisystemic manifestations, or intellectual impairment.

Clinical Presentation: Signs and Symptoms

In the autosomal dominant variety of MC, both sexes are affected with equal frequency. Generalized myotonia is noted from early childhood and is non-progressive. Both action and percussion myotonia are present but vary in intensity from muscle to muscle. In some patients, the myotonia becomes worse during puberty and remits with advancing age. Additionally, exposure to cold, fatigue, inactivity, menstruation, and pregnancy exacerbate the myotonia. Because the myotonia is worse with the initial attempt at movement following a period of rest, patients frequently report feeling stiff and "like a board" on rising from a sustained seated posture. Muscle weakness is not found in the autosomal dominant variety. The most striking physical sign is the generalized muscle hypertrophy, which when severe, gives the patient a Herculean appearance. This enhanced muscle bulk is especially prominent in the gluteal, quadriceps, gastrocnemius, deltoid, biceps and triceps muscles.

Myotonia congenita of autosomal recessive inheritance has a later onset than the dominant type. Two-thirds of these patients are males. Myotonia is more pronounced in this group and in addition to muscle hypertrophy, there is weakness, although mild, in the distal upper and lower extremities. The weakness, unlike the myotonia which may progress until puberty, is non-progressive. (Harper and Johnston, 1972). As in the autosomal dominant variety, exposure to cold and inactivity increases the myotonia.

Myotonia congenita is easily distinguished from the other myotonic disorders. Diffuse muscle hypertrophy and generalized myotonia are unique to MC. Severe muscle weakness and wasting, involvement of other organ systems and endocrine abnormalities are not encountered in MC but they are present in myotonic atrophy. Paramyotonia congenita differs from MC by the absence of muscle hypertrophy and by the characteristic occurrence of myotonia and weakness predominantly on exposure to cold. The myopathy that accompanies hypothyroidism may resemble MyC. However, the latter is characterized by myoedema and elevated CPK levels, neither of which are manifestations of MyC.

Laboratory Studies

Muscle biopsy

Routine microscopic examination of muscle tissue in patients with MC generally reveal no abnormalities. However, histochemical staining has shown a complete absence of type II B fibers in many afflicted individuals (Crews et al, 1976) which can be demonstrated by the reverse ATPase reaction (pH 4.6).

Electromyography

Myotonic discharges are readily demonstrated by EMG studies. These are found in virtually all muscles.

Serum muscle enzymes

Serum levels of muscle enzymes in both forms of MC are normal.

Prognosis and Treatment

The myotonia and muscle hypertrophy of MC persist unchanged throughout the adult life of the patient. Longevity is not shortened by the disease and most patients live normal lives within the limitations imposed by the myotonia.

Individuals with disabling myotonia should be treated with phenytoin (200-400 mg daily), procainamide (1-4 g daily) or quinine (500-1500 mg daily). (Munsat, 1967; Kin and Yamada, 1974). Acetazolamide (250-750 mg daily) also appears to be acceptable therapy for occasional patients with myotonia who are unresponsive to or intolerant of other therapies (Griggs et al, 1978).

PARAMYOTONIA CONGENITA

Paramyotonia congenita (PC) is a rare disorder first recognized by Eulenberg in 1886. Because of its close resemblance to hyperkalemic periodic paralysis, its existence as a distinct entity has been questioned. In Eulenberg's classic description of the disorder, myotonic features were present only under the influence of cold. After the patient warmed up, the myotonic stiffness was fol-

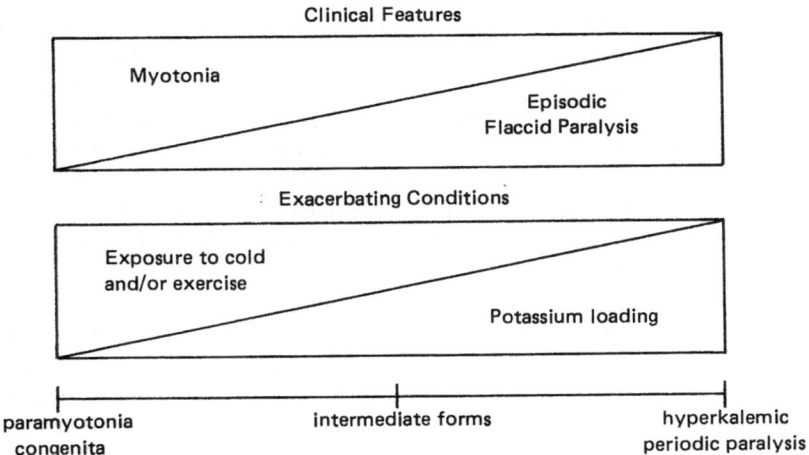

Figure 6-4. Continuous clinical spectrum of the paramyotonic disorders and periodic paralyses.

lowed by a flaccid paralysis of variable duration. Since this initial description, numerous families have been reported with symptoms similar but not identical to those of Eulenberg. Some have described patients with cold-induced myotonia and paradoxical myotonia but without episodic paresis (Brungger and Kaeser, 1977). Others have reported patients whose symptoms were induced by an oral potassium load as well as by exposure to cold (Samaha, 1964). It has thus become evident that paramyotonia congenita and hyperkalemic periodic paralysis (hyper PP) have many features in common and that a variety of intermediate syndromes sharing aspects of both, also exist. Both paramyotonia congenita and hyper PP have autosomal dominant inheritance, myotonia increased by cold, and episodes of flaccid paresis. They differ, however, in that the paralysis in hyper PP is of longer duration.

In addition, the myotonia and paralysis are much more sensitive to oral potassium loading in families with hyper PP than in cases of paramyotonia congenita. Furthermore, paradoxical myotonia, a hallmark of paramyotonia, is not found in hyper PP. More recently, it has been observed that these two entities also differ in their responses to acetazolamide (Riggs et al, 1977). Probably it is best to view these two syndromes as diseases at opposing ends of a continuous spectrum of disorders characterized by myotonia and episodic paresis (see Figure 6-3).

Symptoms of paramyotonia congenita may be noted shortly after birth, but usually become manifest during the first decade of life. Typically, the myotonia is paradoxical, generalized, and markedly increased by cold. Persistent myotonia is present in some patients and is most pronounced in the finger flexors and facial muscles. Occasionally, the extraocular muscles are involved with resultant diplopia. During or after vigorous exercise myotonia develops in previously asymptomatic muscle groups (paradoxical myotonia). Within a few minutes, the diffuse myotonic stiffness is succeeded by a flaccid paresis which may last 15 minutes or longer. This paralysis is most prominent in the lower extremities and cranial musculature. A similar sequence of events can be precipitated by prolonged exposure to cold.

Patients with PC typically complain of painful spasms of the tongue when eating ice cream, and of clumsiness of their hands during the winter. Several have reported near drowning after diving into a cool swimming pool. Most patients, however, learn early in life to avoid prolonged exposures to cold, and they live nearly normal lives. Muscular hypertrophy is not a prominent feature in PC as it is in myotonia congenita. The absence of weakness and multisystemic involvement differentiates the disease from myotonic atrophy. In addition, oral potassium loading usually does not markedly increase symptoms and this helps to differentiate it from typical hyper PP (Baxter and Dyck, 1961; Magee, 1966; Lindberg et al, 1974).

Laboratory Studies

Serum muscle enzymes

Patients with paramyotonia congenita generally have normal levels of CPK and other muscle enzymes.

Electromyography

Typically, patients with paramyotonia congenita show myotonic discharges which increase with repetitive forceful contractions and on cooling, and diminish with warming of the muscles being tested (Burke et al, 1974).

Muscle biopsy

The diagnosis of paramyotonia congenita is a clinical one and muscle biopsy is not helpful in confirming the diagnosis. Changes in muscle tissue in such individuals are generally non-specific.

Cold provocation test

In an individual suspected of having paramyotonia, the abnormality can frequently be brought out by immersing the upper extremity up to the elbow in cold water (10°C) for 30 minutes. Strength and myotonia are then evaluated at 5, 10, 15, and 30 minute intervals. Patients with the disorder will show increased action and percussion myotonia under these conditions.

Prognosis and Treatment

Symptomatic myotonia occurs between the ages of three and ten years, and increases thereafter until puberty. It then gradually diminishes during adult life and occasionally becomes exacerbated during pregnancy. Most patients live relatively normal lives with few limitations. Specific treatment is generally not necessary other than warning the patient of the hazards of prolonged exposure to cold and of vigorous activity. Drug therapy, if required, should be restricted to phenytoin (200-400 mg/day) or procainamide (1-4 g/day) (Munsat, 1967). Acetazolamide should not be used in these patients because it may worsen the paresis (Riggs et al, 1977).

CHAPTER 7

The Periodic Paralysis

HYPOKALEMIC PERIODIC PARALYSIS

Familial hypokalemic periodic paralysis (hypo PP) is a disorder character-ized by proxysmal attacks of flaccid weakness involving the extremities and trunk. Such episodes are usually associated with a decrease in the patient's serum potassium concentration. While the majority of cases are inherited in an autoso-mal dominant fashion, approximately five percent are sporadic.

Until recently there was no effective treatment of the disorder, and afflicted individuals were severely restricted in their activity. However, the drug acetazola-mide has dramatically changed the outlook for these patients and has enabled the majority of them to lead nearly normal lives.

Clinical Presentation: Signs and Symptoms

The episodes of weakness which characterize hypokalemic periodic paraly-sis have their onset in the second decade. Typically they vary in frequency, severity, and duration. Severe attacks begin in the lower extremities, and over a period of hours, spread to involve the muscles of the trunk and upper limbs. At the height of such an attack, the patient is quadriplegic but is able to speak, chew, swallow, and move the eyes. Respiratory function is usually minimally compromised. Attacks last between 12 and 72 hours, with return of strength beginning in the muscle groups that were last affected. Excessive thirst, diapho-resis, oliguria, and obstipation commonly precede and accompany an attack, while diuresis is characteristic of the recovery phase. Attacks may occur as of-ten as one to two per week, or as infrequently as one every few years. Patients may experience minor episodes of weakness restricted to the proximal muscle groups of the lower extremities.

Examination of patients during a severe attack most frequently reveals a flaccid quadriplegia with absent tendon reflexes. Affected muscles are electrically and mechanically inexcitable. The preservation of function of the facial oropharyngeal and ocular muscles is striking. Between episodes there are no neurologic abnormalities; however, after a number of years, such patients may develop permanent proximal weakness resembling the limb-girdle dystrophies (Pearson, 1964; Dyken et al, 1969). This fixed proximal myopathy usually does not appear earlier than five years from the time of onset of the disorder.

Affected individuals soon discover that while most of the attacks are unpredictable in their occurrence, certain activities commonly precipitate such episodes. These include heavy exercise followed by rest, excessive carbohydrate intake, alcohol overindulgence, stress, trauma, and cold. In many instances, an incipient attack may be relieved, postponed, or prevented by mild exercise.

During a bout of weakness, the serum potassium level is usually low and less than 2.5 mEq/liter. The drop in the serum potassium precedes the weakness and the level returns to normal prior to clinical recovery of the patient (Gordon et al, 1970). Weakness, however, may be present even when the serum potassium level is only slightly below normal. Accompanying the reduction in potassium are electrocardiographic changes compatible with hypokalemia, including T wave flattening, prominent U waves, and prolonged PR and QT intervals.

Hypokalemic periodic paralysis may rarely occur in association with thyrotoxicosis, or secondary to urinary or gastrointestinal potassium wasting (see Table 7-1).

Initially, patients with periodic paralysis are commonly misdiagnosed as hysterics or malingerers. This is understandable when one is confronted with a patient who several hours ago was perfectly normal and is now unable to move from the neck down. The striking preservation of mental function, of cranial and respiratory musculature, as well as the absence of any pain or antecedent trauma, further mislead the unwary examiner into believing that this is a functional illness. It is only after the patient is examined and the marked hypotonia and hyporeflexia elicited that an organic illness is considered. Other neuromuscular disorders, including Guillain-Barré syndrome (GBS), acute intermittent porphyria (AIP), myasthenia gravis (MG), tick paralysis, and botulism may present as a rapidly evolving symmetric paresis (see Figure 1-1). In the analysis of such a patient, several important clinical features are helpful, including the presence or absence of autonomic dysfunction and cranial nerve abnormalities. Involvement of the autonomic nervous system commonly occurs with GBS, AIP and botulism, while cranial nerve impairment is prominent with MG and botulism. Neither autonomic nor cranial nerve dysfunction occurs with the periodic paralysis. However, to further clarify the diagnosis, laboratory studies (especially EMG) are usually needed.

Table 7-1.   Secondary Hypokalemic Periodic Paralysis

Urinary potassium wasting
hyperaldosteronism
renal tubular acidosis
Fanconi syndrome
thiazide therapy

Gastrointestinal potassium wasting
sprue
villous adenoma of the rectum
laxative abuse
prolonged vomiting
barium carbonate poisoning

Laboratory Studies

Serum muscle enzymes

Creatine phosphokinase levels may be elevated during and immediately following an episode of weakness. Between attacks, however, serum muscle enzyme levels are normal.

Electrodiagnostic tests

During a spontaneous or induced episode of weakness, the muscle fibers become electrically inexcitable. As the attack progresses, the evoked motor response of affected muscles shows decreasing amplitude, and finally no response can be elicited. When the EMG needle is inserted in the paralyzed muscle, there is little or no insertional activity. Such findings are not observed in MG, botulism, GBS, AIP, tick paralysis, or hysteria.

It is of interest that prolonged stimulation of a paralyzed muscle may sometimes result in complete recovery of the evoked response and clinical strength. Cessation of the stimulus is followed by an immediate return of the paralysis. This is analogous to the clinical observation that moderate physical activity wards off an impending attack. Between attacks, electrodiagnostic testing may uncover "myopathic" features in proximal muscle groups (i.e., BSAPP pattern).

Muscle biopsy

Vacuoles in otherwise near normal muscle fibers characterize the biopsy findings in the hypo PP. These vacuoles are present in both ictal and interictal specimens (see Figure 7-1). In addition, tubular aggregates may be observed in type II fibers. At the subcellular level, these vacuoles are actually dilatations of the terminal cisternae and transverse tubules (Dubowitz and Brooke, 1973).

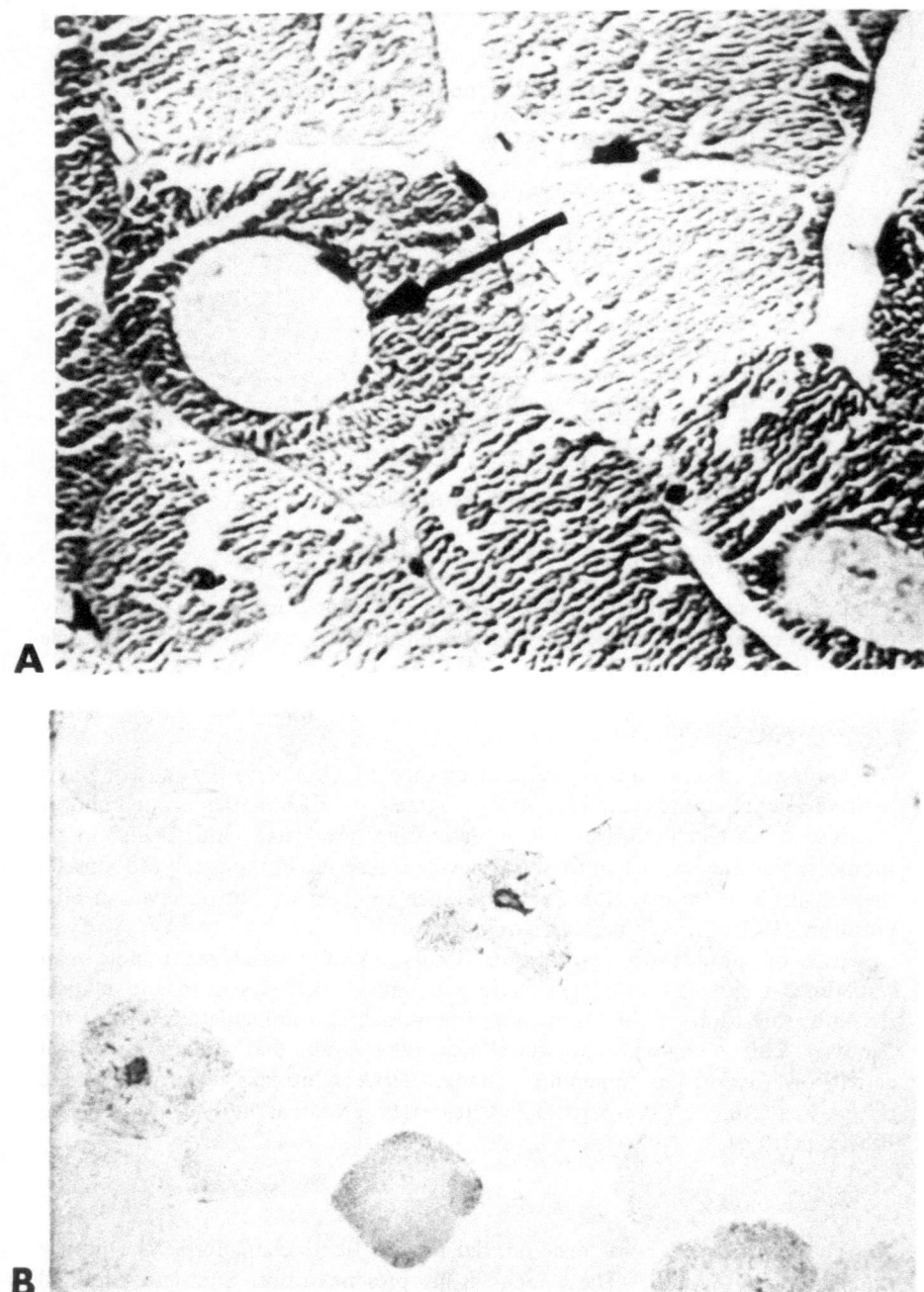

Figure 7-1. Muscle biopsy—hypokalemic periodic paralysis. (A) Note the single smooth round vacuoles that are characterisitc of hypo PP. (B) Note the single central vacuoles as well as the tubular aggregates in this biopsy specimen from a patient with hypo PP

Other tests

Since patients do not always come to the attention of a physician during an attack, it may be necessary to use provocative measures to make the diagnosis. The usual method is to administer 100 g of glucose by mouth and 20 units of insulin subcutaneously. Potassium levels are drawn at 20-minute intervals and evaluation of the patient's strength determined at the time of each blood sample. A clinical attack may occur at any time and may take as long as six hours after the challenge to develop. A clear-cut episode of weakness is diagnostic, but if no weakness occurs, it is imperative to be certain that the serum potassium has dropped to at least 2.5 mEq/liter for the test to be considered an adequate challenge.

Pathophysiology

The primary defect in hypo PP appears to be related to the abnormal permeability and conducting properties of the muscle fiber membrane and its components (sarcoplasmic reticulum and transverse tubules) (Layzer 1982). Acute episodes of weakness are accompanied by shifts of potassium, sodium and H_2O from the extracellular fluid to the interior of the muscle fibers. Exactly why these changes occur and how they produce paresis is unknown, but it has been suggested that such shifts produce a depolarizing block of the muscle fiber membrane thus rendering it inexcitable (Viskoper et al, 1973). Loss of extracellular water with a subsequent fall in plasma volume could explain the observed oliguria and thirst that frequently accompany the episodic paresis.

It has further been proposed that the deranged electrolyte and water concentrations within the muscle fiber ultimately lead to dilatation of the transverse tubules and vacuole formation. Such distended tubules are unable to release calcium effectively in response to muscle action potentials and therefore, despite intact contractile elements, the fiber becomes functionally paralyzed (Engel and Lambert, 1969; Kao and Gordon, 1977). This mechanism could explain the progressive myopathy which develops in many of the patients with longstanding hypo PP.

Treatment

The acute episodes of weakness are most effectively treated with oral potassium salts (20 to 100 mEq) (Griggs, 1977). If the oral route cannot be used, potassium chloride can be administered slowly intravenously (60 to 80 mEq/ liter).

Acetazolamide is the agent of choice for prophylactic treatment of attacks. Previously, low carbohydrate diets, potassium supplements, and spironolactone (Poskanzer and Kerr, 1961) were used but failed to prevent attacks effectively. On the other hand, clinical trials using acetazolamide (125 to 1000 mg/day) have shown that the drug dramatically reduces 'the frequency, severity, and duration of attacks. (Griggs et al, 1970; Griggs 1977). An additional benefit of daily therapy with acetazolamide is an apparent reversal of the chronic inter-ictal weakness. The response to the drug is usually prompt, with attack frequency decreasing within 24 hours of initiation of therapy. Patients do not become refractory to acetazolamide.

Exactly how the drug produces beneficial effects is uncertain. Neither its ability to inhibit carbonic anhydrase nor its kaluretic effect adequately accounts for its therapeutic action. It appears, however, that the metabolic acidosis induced by the drug may be the basis of its beneficial effects (Viskoper et al, 1973; Vroom et al, 1975). The induced acidosis reduces the entry of potassium into muscle fibers thus opposing the pathological shift of this ion during an attack.

Chronic therapy with acetazolamide may be complicated by the development of paresthesias and/or renal calculi. For this reason, patients taking the drug should be instructed to maintain a high fluid intake and obtain periodic abdominal x-rays. If the patient cannot tolerate acetazolamide, dichlorophenamide (50 mg twice daily) may be a suitable alternative (Dalakas and Engel, 1983).

HYPERKALEMIC PERIODIC PARALYSIS
(ADYNAMIA EPISODICA HEREDITARIA)

A rare familial disorder characterized by episodic weakness and elevated levels of plasma potassium was first described by Gamstorp in 1956. She called this entity adynamia episodica hereditaria. Subsequently, a number of cases were reported similar to those described by Gamstorp except that many of these exhibited cold-sensitive myotonia in addition to paroxysmal bouts of weakness. Thus the close relationship of this disorder to paramyotonia congenita of von Eulenberg became evident (see Chapter 6). Additional case material revealed that the serum potassium concentration may remain normal during some of the attacks of paresis, and that the response of the patient to oral potassium loading rather than the absolute plasma potassium level best characterized the disorder (Griggs, 1977). Because of the observations many now consider normokalemic periodic paralysis a subgroup of hyperkalemic periodic paralysis and not a distinct entity.

Clinical Presentation: Signs and Symptoms

Hyperkalemic periodic paralysis (hyper PP) is an autosomal dominant disorder that has its onset most commonly in the first decade of life. As in hypokalemic periodic paralysis, attacks vary in frequency, duration, and severity. Patients may experience daily bouts of weakness or episodes may occur as infrequently as one or two per year. A typical attack begins with a stiff, heavy, or tingly feeling in the lower extremities. This is soon followed by weakness in these limbs. The paresis may remain restricted to this area or it may spread to involve muscles of the trunk, upper extremities, and neck. Cranial musculature is generally spared and respiratory function only minimally compromised. The duration of an attack is shorter than those in the hypokalemic form, with most of the attacks abating in one-half to four hours.

Myotonia may or may not be a prominent component of the disorder; however, when present, it may assume a number of different patterns. Some patients have asymptomatic (percussion) myotonia which then becomes symptomatic during an attack. Others experience myotonia only during an attack, and still others have episodic myotonia without weakness (Layzer et al, 1967).

When myotonia is present, it most frequently involves the extraocular muscles (the eyes becoming "stuck" when the patient attempts to gaze shift) and the facial muscles (with the patient unable to open the eyes after forced closure). Occasionally the oropharyngeal muscles become myotonic with resultant dysphagia.

Most patients with the disorder exhibit elevated levels of the serum potassium in association with their episodes of weakness. During this time, the potassium concentration is found to be 2 to 4 mEq/liter above the normal base line value. Some patients have attacks in which the plasma potassium level is normal but this occurrence may be a result of sampling venous blood from areas not affected by the particular episode.

Attacks may be provoked by exercise followed by rest, exposure to cold, sleep, anesthesia, fasting, emotional stress, and oral potassium loading. They may at times be warded off by light exercise and/or a high carbohydrate meal.

Examination of such patients during a bout of weakness reveals flaccid paresis of affected muscles and diminished tendon reflexes. As already discussed, myotonia may or may not be present. Between attacks, patients may exhibit some degree of myotonia and/or mild proximal muscle weakness.

During childhood, attacks are more frequent and tend to increase at the time of pubescence. After age 30, there seems to be a considerable reduction in the number of episodes (Gamstorp et al, 1957). As with cases of the hypokalemic variety, patients with hyperkalemic periodic paralysis may be mistakenly accused of malingering or misdiagnosed as Guillain-Barré syndrome or as other entities capable of producing a rapidly ascending quadriparesis (Figure

1-1). In this situation, EMG studies are most helpful (see discussion of hypo-kalemic periodic paralysis).

Laboratory Studies

Muscle biopsy

Abnormalities of muscle tissue morphology in patients with adynamia are identical to those found in hypokalemic periodic paralysis.

Electromyography

During a paretic episode the muscles are electrically inexcitable. With needle examination of the muscle, one is struck by the markedly reduced insertional activity.

Serum muscle enzymes

The serum creatine phosphokinase level may be elevated during or immediately following a bout of paresis, but otherwise muscle enzyme concentration are normal.

Other

The diagnosis of hyper PP is established by finding an elevated serum potassium level during an attack of weakness and/or by reproducing such attacks with an oral potassium challenge (Gamstorp et al, 1957). Continuous ECG monitoring of the patient is mandatory when such a challenge test is performed.

Pathophysiology

Paretic episodes and myotonia in adynamia are probably related to abnormal muscle membrane function and disordered ion transport across the sarcolemma. Studies have demonstrated that the resting membrane potential in hyper PP is decreased (approximately -65 mV) and that during an attack, the membrane potential remains in a fixed depolarized state (Bradley, 1969; Brooks, 1969). It appears that in these patients the low resting membrane potential is the result of failure of the sodium-potassium pump mechanism. When stressed (i.e., exercise, fasting, and potassium intake), this compromised system cannot maintain the already reduced resting membrane potential above threshold and the result is a sustained depolarization.

Treatment

Acute episodes of weakness may at times respond to high carbohydrate foods. More severe attacks, however, require intravenous glucose and insulin. Recently it has been shown that inhalation of salbutamol, a beta-adrenergic agonist, at the time of an attack may abort the episode or at least decrease its severity (Wang and Clausen, 1976).

Chronic therapy to prevent attacks consists of either daily thiazide diuretics or acetazolamide. Thiazides may be preferable to acetazolamide since they are at least as effective and are associated with fewer side effects (Griggs, 1977). Dietary management consisting of high carbohydrate and low sodium intake has also reportedly been effective (Brillman and Pincus, 1973).

NORMOKALEMIC PERIODIC PARALYSIS

Normokalemic periodic paralysis (normo PP) is an autosomal dominantly inherited disease in which the serum potassium level remains unchanged during paroxysmal episodes of paresis. It is difficult to know whether this disorder is an entity in its own right or whether the reports cited are merely atypical variants of hyperkalemic periodic paralysis. Most authorities feel that there is a significant number of dissimilarities between norms PP and other periodic paralyses to justify its existence as a distinct nosologic entity.

Clinical Presentation: Signs and Symptoms

Typically the disorder has its onset in the first decade of life. Attacks occur every few months and vary in duration from minutes to days. Mild attacks remain restricted to the extensor muscle groups of the upper and lower limbs. More severe episodes result in a flaccid quadriplegia without significant respiratory impairment. There is no bowel, bladder, or sensory dysfunction. Myotonia, so prominent in the hyperkalemic variety is not found in these patients. Facial musculature and other bulbar structures are seldom affected.

Between attacks, patients may exhibit mild weakness in the extensors of the extremities and in calf muscles. In addition, hypertrophy of the triceps and gastroc-nemis muscles is noted in a significant number of patients.

Episodes of paresis may be induced by alcohol intoxication, over sleeping, and mental stress. Rest after exertion, however, is the most common precipitating factor (Poskanzer and Kerr, 1961).

During paretic attacks, the serum potassium levels remain unchanged. Furthermore, attacks are not induced by making these patients either hypo- or hyperkalemic (Meyers et al, 1972).

Table 7-2. Summary of the Periodic Paralyses

Type	Inheritance	Age of Onset	Attacks Provoked by:	Attacks: Frequency	Attacks: Duration	Attacks: Symptoms	Serum K^+	Treatment
hypokalemic	autosomal dominant	second decade	rest after exercise high carbohydrate intake alcohol intoxication cold exposure	2/week to less than 1/year	12 to 72 hours	flaccid weakness in lower extremities which ascends-thirst, oliguria, and diaphoresis	usually less than 2.5 mEq / liter	KCl acetazolamide low carbohydrate diet
hyperkalemic	autosomal dominant	first decade	rest after exercise fasting cold exposure oral KCl	daily to 1-2/year	30 minutes to 4 hours	tingling in lower extremities followed by ascending flaccid quadriplegia myotonia	usually greater than 5.5 mEq / liter but may be normal	glucose-insulin insulin salbutamol thiazides acetazolamide
normokalemic	autosomal dominant	first decade	rest after exercise over sleeping alcohol intoxication	3 to 6 per year	minutes to days	weakness of extensor muscle groups progressing to quadriplegia	usually normal	NaCl

Laboratory Studies

Serum muscle enzymes

Serum muscle enzymes may be mildly elevated during and between attacks.

Muscle biopsy

Muscle biopsy in these patients shows central vacuolization of type II fibers some of which contain PAS positive material (Meyers, et al, 1972).

Electromyography

Electrodiagnostic testing during a paretic episode characteristically shows numerous low amplitude, short duration, polyphasic potentials (Poskanzer and Kerr, 1961).

Treatment

Oral or intravenous sodium chloride is the agent of choice for treating acute attacks. Prophylactic therapy with alpha fluorohydrocortisone and acetazolamide may be effective (Poskanzer and Kerr, 1961). Thiazides, useful as a therapy for hyper PP, are ineffective for normokalemic periodic paralysis.

CHAPTER 8

Inflammatory Myopathies

VIRAL MYOSITIS

With certain viral infections, myalgias may be prominent. The muscle pain and tenderness tend to involve the lower extremities (especially the calves) and are generally short-lived. Infections with enterovirus (coxsackie, poliovirus, and echovirus) and influenza virus (Ruff and Secrist, 1982) are most commonly associated with this syndrome. In one variety (Bronholm disease) there is selective involvement of the diaphragm and intercostal muscles, and pleurodynia is prominent. Coxsackie type B is the culprit in most cases.

Children are much more susceptible to these illnesses than are adults. Muscle biopsy has been performed in some instances and variable necrosis and inflammatory cell infiltration have been found.

TRICHINOSIS

Trichinella infection in humans is found everywhere from the artic region to the tropics. While the incidence of the disease in the United States has diminished substantially, it still remains the most common helminthic infestation of man. Trichinosis is primarily a disease of humans and pigs. Human infection, which in the vast majority of cases is subclinical, results from eating infected, inadequately cooked pork or pork products. Occasional outbreaks have followed the ingestion of bear or walrus meat. The infected meat (skeletal muscle) contains the encysted larval stage of the nematode Trichinella spiralis. In the small intestine (jejunum) the larvae are liberated by digestion of the cyst wall, become attached to the mucosa, and grow. Within two days they become sexually mature and copulate. The males die, but the females give birth to living larvae (up to 1,500 per fertilized female) that are deposited directly into surrounding venules and lacteals. The larvae disseminate systemically and settle preferentially

in skeletal muscles where they encyst. These cysts then grow and eventually cal-
cify (within 6 to 18 months). Larvae carried to other sites (i.e., central nervous
system and myocardium) generally do not encyst but nevertheless are capable of
producing significant dysfunction at these locales. For completion of the cycle,
encysted larvae must be ingested by a suitable host. The practice of feeding uncooked, infected pork scraps to swine serves to perpetuate hog infection. The
life cycle of Trichinella spiralis is summarized in Figure 8-1.

Clinical Presentation: Signs and Symptoms

Trichinosis varies in its manifestations from asymptomatic cases to severe
fulminating infections resulting in death. In symptomatic cases, the major organ
systems involved include the skeletal muscles and, less often, the central nervous
system and myocardium. Symptomatology can be divided into three phases:
intestinal, migratory, and encystment (Gray et al, 1962). The intestinal stage
occurs within 48 hours of ingestion of the infected meat. It is characterized by
fever, diarrhea, abdominal pain, anorexia, nausea, and vomiting, all of which are
self-limiting. During this stage, larvae are penetrating the small bowel mucosa.
Day 7 to 14, the migratory phase, is marked by the appearance of periorbital
edema, subungual splinter hemorrhages, and urticaria. Signs of a meningo-encephalitis including headache, nuchal rigidity, delirium and lethargy may be present at this time. These signs are believed to result from a hypersensitivity reaction.

The final stage of the illness is characterized by encystment of larvae in
skeletal muscle tissue and occasionally by signs indicative of central nervous
system and/or myocardial involvement. During this time, there is severe muscle
pain, weakness, and diminished deep tendon reflexes. The most frequently afflicted muscles are the tongue, masseter, extra-ocular, diaphragm, deltoid and
intercostal muscles (Plorde 1977). Difficulty with chewing, dysphagia, trismus,
diplopia, and painful eye and respiratory movement are frequent complains.
Focal neurologic signs occur in five to twenty percent of cases (Gray et al,
1962). Hemiplegia, dysphasia, cerebellar ataxia, seizures, cranial nerve palsies
(VI, VII), and cavernous sinus thrombosis (Barr, 1966) may appear. Evidence of
focal CNS damage is an ominous sign and carries a 40 percent mortality (Aita,
1973). Unlike the meningo-encephalitis, focal neurologic signs are attributed to
larvae occluding small vessels, thus producing infarction, hemorrhage, and
edema.

Cardiac involvement, when it occurs, does so during the third week of the
disease. Evidence of myocardial invasion is heralded by electrocardiographic
changes including T wave flattening and inversion, conduction defects, and arrhythmias. In many instances a florid myocarditis with congestive heart failure
follows.

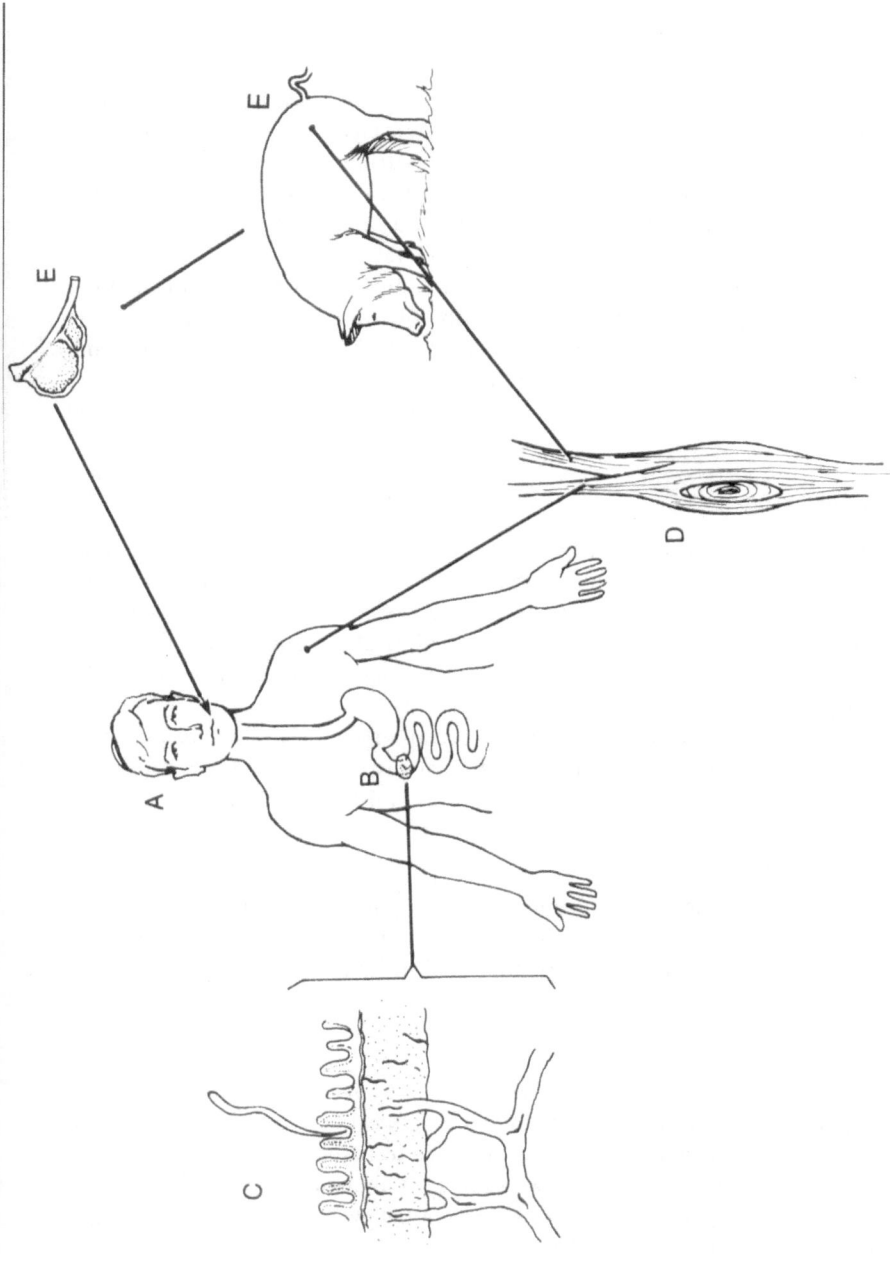

Figure 8-1. Life cycle of Trichinella spiralis. Man (A) eats infected pork (E). Larvae reach jejunum (B) where they mature, mate, and deposit live larvae into surrounding blood vessels and lacteals (C). Larvae then migrate and encyst in skeletal muscle (D). The cycle is perpetuated in hogs by the practice of feeding uncooked pork scaps to these animals.

Laboratory Studies

Serum muscle enzymes and other blood tests

Serum muscle enzymes, including creatinine phosphokinase, and transaminases, and aldolase are usually elevated and often eight to ten times above expected values. Characteristic of the illness is a striking peripheral eosinophilia which becomes apparent during the second week of infection, peaks during the fourth week, and gradually subsides over several months. A precipitous fall in the eosinophil count may be the harbinger of a fatal termination.

Serologic tests for trichinosis, including the precipitin complement-fixation, bentonite-flocculation, and fluorescent antibody tests, become positive by the third week of infection. These tests are most valuable if they are negative initially and then turn positive or if there is a change in titer. Larvae are found so rarely in blood and spinal fluid that the attempt to find them is hardly justified (Most, 1978).

Muscle biopsy

Muscle biopsy is the definitive diagnostic procedure. Since larvae are most numerous at the sites of muscular attachments to tendons, it is wise to choose a specimen at such a locale. The tissue is then pressed between glass slides and examined microscopically. Larvae appear as elliptical structures with thick capsules. Surrounding the cysts may be an inflammatory reaction consisting of mononuclear cells and eosinophils (see Figure 8-2).

If the compression technique fails to reveal larvae, it is recommended that a portion of the biopsy be digested in artificial gastric juice that will permit exposure of the more deeply encysted larvae (Beck and Davies, 1976).

Electromyography

Electromyographic studies during the acute phase of the illness commonly show fibrillations, sharp waves, and marked diminution in the amplitude and duration of the motor unit action potentials (BSAPP pattern).

Pathogenesis

The clinical manifestations of trichinosis result from a combination of mechanical and allergic factors. Muscle pain and weakness, and focal neurologic signs are largely the result of mechanical damage to tissue and of the obstruction of blood vessels. Other manifestations such as the meningo-encephalitis, angioneurotic edema, urticaria, and hemorrhages are believed to be secondary to immunologic phenomena. Both digestive tract end products and genital secretions of Trichinello spiralis have been shown to be strongly antigenic.

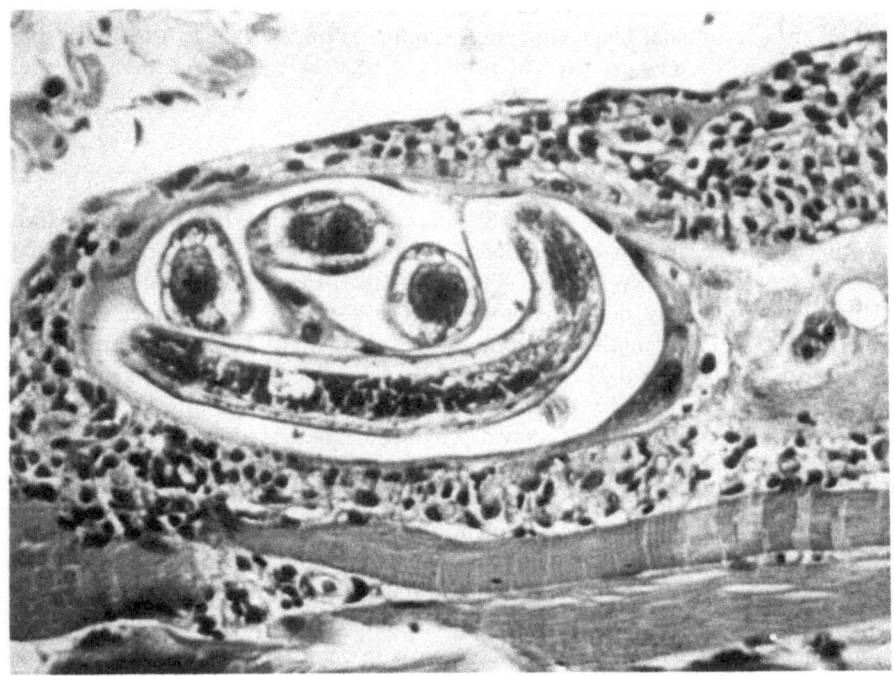

Figure 8-2. Muscle biopsy—trichinosis. An encysted larva is seen at the top of the figure.

Prognosis and Treatment

Prognosis in trichinosis is determined by the degree of infestation and whether or not there is CNS and/or myocardial involvement. When the latter organ systems are involved, mortality is high despite appropriate therapy (Kramer and Aita, 1972). Adequate treatment includes administration of the antihelminthic "thiabendazole" and steroids. The recommended dose of thiabendazole is 25-50 mg/kg/day for seven to ten days. The drug not only destroys encapsulated larvae in skeletal muscle but also interferes with larval reproduction and promotes expulsion of Trichinella spiralis from the gut. Thus it is effective also as a prophylactic agent in patients with a known recent exposure to trichinous meat. Abrupt dissolution of the larvae with massive release of protein breakdown products can cause a Herxheimer-like reaction, and for this reason corticosteroids (40-60 mg of prednisone or its equivalent) should be administered concomitantly (Davis et al, 1976).

Prevention of the disease can only be accomplished by adequate cooking of all pork products. Meat inspection stamps do not pertain to trichinosis and their presence is no guarantee of protection against contracting the infection.

CYSTICERCOSIS

Infestation by the larval or bladder-worm stage of the pork tapeworm Taenia solium results in cysticerocosis. While the illness is rare in the United States, it is common in parts of Europe, Africa, Central and South America. Humans are the only definitive hosts for the adult tapeworm which measures six to ten feet in length and contains approximately 1,000 segments called "proglottids", (Figure 8-3). The head of the worm or scolex contains four suckers and two rows of hooks that help anchor it to the host's intestinal mucosa. With maturation of the adult, gravid proglottids are passed in the feces, each of which may contain up to 30,000 ova (Jacob and Mathew, 1968). The coprophagous habits of pigs lead to heavy infection with ova. In the intermediate host, whether it be a hog or a human, ova develop into oncospheres that claw their way through the gut wall and penetrate lymphatics and blood vessels. After traveling through the circulation, they come to rest in various tissues including skeletal muscle, nervous and subcutaneous tissue. Here they develop into the cysticercus stage. Man then ingests infected, improperly cooked pork and the cycle is perpetuated.

Humans may serve as the intermediate hosts for Taenia solium and it is when this occurs, that symptoms develop. Man becomes the intermediate host by ingesting food or drink contaminated by human feces containing ova, or by auto-infection resulting from regurgitation of ripe proglottids from the upper small intestine into the stomach. Such auto-infection occurs in 25 percent of cases.

Fully developed cysticerci are small (5 X 10 mm) bladder-shaped structures that contain an inverted scolex (Figure 8-3). Living cysts are small and impalpable. When they die after three to five years, they swell and become tense with fluid. At this stage they may be clinically palpable in subcutaneous tissue and, less often, in muscle.

Clinical Presentation: Signs and Symptoms

Cysticercosis in man most commonly presents with epilepsy and/or hydrocephalus. Muscle involvement is common, but usually clinically silent. When extensive invasion of the musculoskeletal system occurs, massive symmetrical enlargement of muscles resembling primary muscle disease is the usual mode of presentation. This striking pseudohypertrophy is most prominent in the calves,

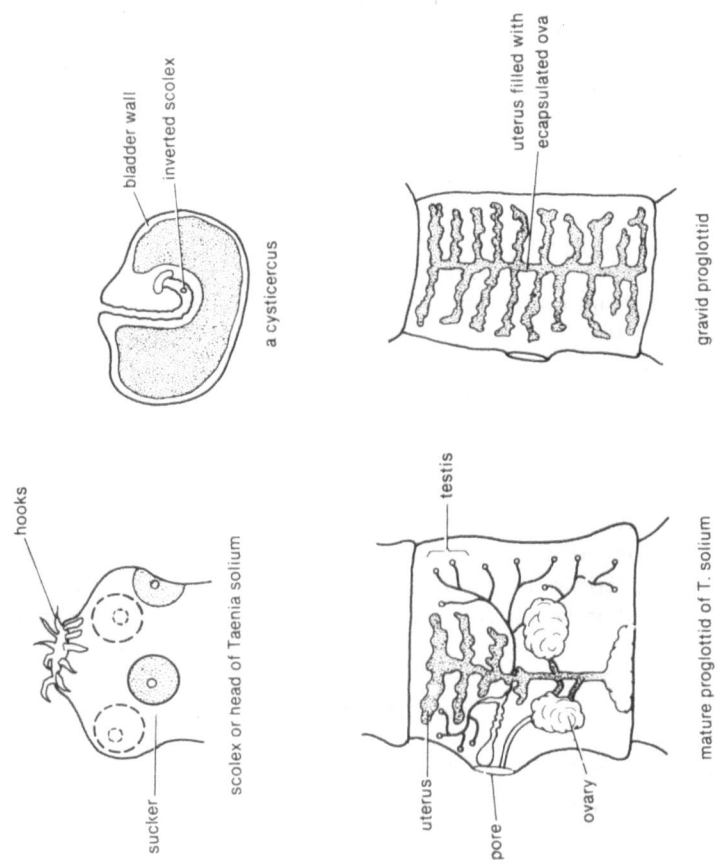

Figure 8-3. Anatomy of Taenia solium.

hip girdle, shoulder girdle, proximal upper arms and thighs. Pain and weakness are minimal and may be entirely absent.

The absence of cramps and myotonia differentiates the illness from myotonia congenita, while the later age of onset, rapidity of development of the hypertrophy, absence of weakness, and negative family history help distinguish it from muscular dystrophy. Disorders of glycogen metabolism and hypothyroidism may produce similarly enlarged, bulky msucles but these disorders are easily distinguished by appropriate laboratory studies.

Palpable subcutaenous nodules are present in over 60 percent of cases and are important for making a tissue diagnosis. Neurologic manifestations include seizures of all types, focal motor and sensory deficits, and hydrocephalus with its sequelae. The syndrome of spinal cord compression may rarely be the result of cysticerci in the spinal subarachnoid space.

Laboratory Studies

Cysticercosis involving the musculoskeletal system generally does not produce elevated serum muscle enzyme levels. A peripheral eosinophilia is present only in about ten percent of cases. Complement fixation tests for Taenia solium are diagnostic if strongly positive (greater than 1:16), but false positives occur with multiple sclerosis, neurosyphilis and some brain tumors (Hoffman and Cuthrie, 1975). Soft tissue x-rays of the limbs reveal intramuscular calcifications in many instances and are often the first clue in an unsuspected case.

Diagnosis is usually easily established by examining the subcutaneous nodules. Frequently, when the overlying skin is incised, cysts pour out and the diagnosis is obvious. Intramuscular cysts, when examined microscopically, contain the characteristic scolex of Taenia solium. These cysts may be surrounded by a mild inflammatory reaction with eosinophils and lymphocytes predominating.

Pathogenesis

Live larvae in muscle are well tolerated by the host and may exist here for several years before producing symptoms. When these larvae finally die, the cysts swell and at this stage, muscle hypertrophy, occasionally accompanied by pain, occurs. Since at least some of the intramuscular cysts are surrounded by an inflammatory exudate, an allergic reaction to foreign larval breakdown products has been implicated as a contributing factor to muscle symptomatology (Sawhney et al, 1976).

Prognosis and Treatment

Although the adult pork tapeworm in the intestine produces few, if any, symptoms, treatment is recommended to prevent auto-infection with ova. Niclosamide (2 g chewed thoroughly in a single dose) is the drug of choice (Beck and Davies, 1976). It is important to avoid nausea and vomiting at this time in order to prevent reverse peristalsis and introduction of gravid proglottids into the stomach. Treatment for cysticercosis is unsatisfactory. Seizures can be controlled with standard anti-convulsants (diaphenylhydantoin and phenobarbital). If signs of an obstructive hydrocephalus develop, neurosurgical intervention may be necessary. Recently a new drug (praziquantel) has been used in the treatment of patients with neurocysticercosis and the results are promising (Botero and Castaño, 1982).

POLYMYOSITIS AND DERMATOMYOSITIS

Polymyositis is an inflammatory myopathy of unknown cause. When a characteristic skin rash accompanies the muscle disorder, the term dermatomyositis is applied. While the disease can begin at virtually any age, 60 percent of cases occur after the age of 40 (DeVere and Bradley, 1975). A variety of collagen vascular diseases including rheumatoid arthritis, systemic lupus erythematosus, progressive systemic sclerosis, polyarteritis nodosa, and Sjögren's syndrome may be complicated by the development of polymyositis. Certain drugs, most notably penicillamine (Schraeder et al, 1972) may produce a similar form of myopathy.

The association of polymyositis-dermatomyositis with neoplasia is well known. The exact incidence of occult malignancies in this disorder varies from 6.7 percent (Christianson et al, 1956) to 34.3 percent (Arundell et al, 1960). A recent study (Devere and Bradley, 1975) found that neoplasia is much more common with dermatomyositis than with polymyositis (29 percent as compared to 8 percent), and that males over 40 years of age with dermatomyositis have a particularly high incidence of malignancy (66 percent). The frequency of tumor types in these patients is outlined in Table 8-1.

It is evident that the distribution of tumors in these disorders differs significantly from that in the general population, with tumors of the ovary and stomach found more commonly and colorectal malignancies under-represented. Barnes (1976) in her review found that in the majority of cases tumor and myopathy presented within a relatively short time of one another (less than one year). It is of note that the disease in childhood, unlike that in adulthood, is idiopathic and rarely associated with an underlying malignancy.

Table 8-1. Comparison of the Most Frequent Tumors Associated with Dermatomyositis and Their Frequency in the General Population (Barnes, 1976)

Tumor Site	Percentage of Cancer in Population	Percentage of Cancer in Dermatomyositis
breast	13.7	17.8
lung	12.6	16.1
ovary	2.6	8.5
stomach	3.5	8.1
colon	15.1	6.6
uterus	7.0	6.6
nasopharyngeal	—	5.8
lymphoma	4.2	5.0
prostate	8.2	3.9

The onset of the disease may be acute or insidious with proximal limb girdle weakness and easy fatigability among the earliest complaints. The weakness is generally symmetric and spreads to involve the neck flexors and occasionally the distal musculature as well. Bulbar muscles may be involved, with 30 percent of patients reporting some degree of dysphagia. Ptosis and diplopia rarely, if ever, occur. Respiratory impairment secondary to intercostal muscle disease is seen in less than five percent of cases: Cardiac muscle is generally spared.

Muscle atrophy does not occur until late so that early in the disease, muscle strength is diminished out of proportion to the degree of wasting. Deep tendon reflexes are normal and sensory abnormalities are not present.

A prominent complaint of the patient is of muscle pain and aching. This is most severe in the shoulders, trapezial ridges, and upper arms, and increases when movements are attempted. With dermatomyositis a classic skin rash appears characterized by a lilac discoloration over the malar aspect of the face and eyelids (heliotrope) with periorbital edema. A scaly erythematous dermatitis over the dorsi of the hands, knuckles, elbows, malleoli of the ankles, neck and upper torso (Gottron's sign) may also be evident.

Additionally, 50 percent of patients with polymyositis-dermatomyositis exhibit Raynaud's phenomenon and one-third will have diffuse joint complaints.

Laboratory Studies

The differential diagnosis of the patient with painful proximal weakness includes non-infectious and infectious inflammatory myopathies (i.e., viral myositis and trichinosis), eosinophilic fasciitis (EF) and Eaton-Lambert syndrome (ELS) (see Table 1-6). Laboratory studies help to differentiate these entities. In trichinosis and EF there is a striking peripheral eosinophilia in most cases. This is not found in polymyositis. Serum CPK levels, if elevated, make Eaton-Lambert syndrome and EF unlikely. Electrodiagnostic studies are helpful in further excluding ELS as a diagnostic possibility.

If the proximal weakness is relatively non-painful, then a dystrophy, endocrine myopathy, sarcoid myopathy, myasthenia gravis, adult acid maltase deficiency, and muscle carnitine deficiency should be considered. In addition, spinal muscular atrophies and proximal neuropathies may present in this manner. Muscle biopsy and electrodiagnostic tests are neeed to evaluate these entities.

Serum muscle enzymes

Serum levels of sarcoplasmic enzymes are generally elevated and serial determinations of these enzymes are of great value in assessing the efficacy of treatment and activity of the disease. Creatine phosphokinase is elevated in approximately 60 to 70 percent of cases. Aldolase, transaminases, and lactic acid dehydrogenase are similarly increased in the serum. It is important to keep in mind that these enzyme values are not infallible guidelines regarding activity of the inflammatory process, and a normal CPK does not by itself exclude polymyositis as the diagnosis. This is especially true in the childhood cases where the CPK is frequently normal.

Electromyography

Electromyographic studies are abnormal in almost 90 percent of cases (DeVere and Bradley, 1975). The classic triad of EMG changes in polymyositis include:

1. short, small polyphasic motor unit potentials (BSAPP pattern);
2. fibrillations, positive sharp waves, and insertional irritability;
3. bizarre high frequency repetitive discharges.

Serial EMG's are helpful in determining response to therapy and in foreseeing a relapse. The earliest EMG sign of improvement is the disappearance of the fibrillation potentials and relapse is often heralded by their reappearance (Bohan and Peters, 1975).

Muscle biopsy

Light microscopic examination of muscle tissue in polymyositis-dermatomyositis is invaluable and, in most cases, is virtually diagnostic. Classically, one observes muscle fiber destruction with regeneration, and pervascular and interstitial inflammation (predominantly lymphocytic) (see Figure 8-4). In addition, positive staining of the connective tissue with the alkaline phosphatase reaction and fiber atrophy in a perifascicular distribution are characteristic features. Some or

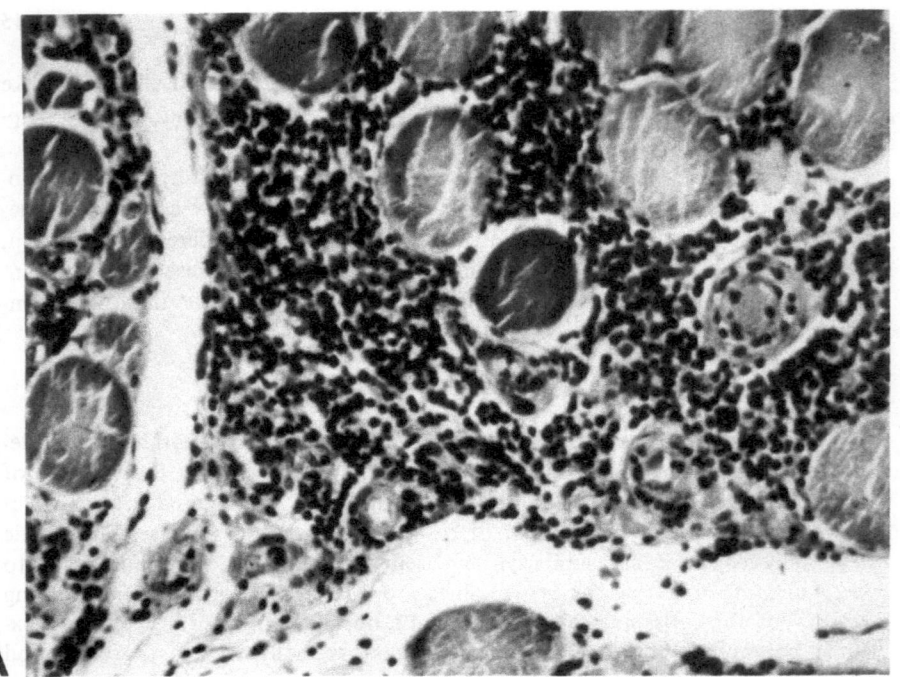

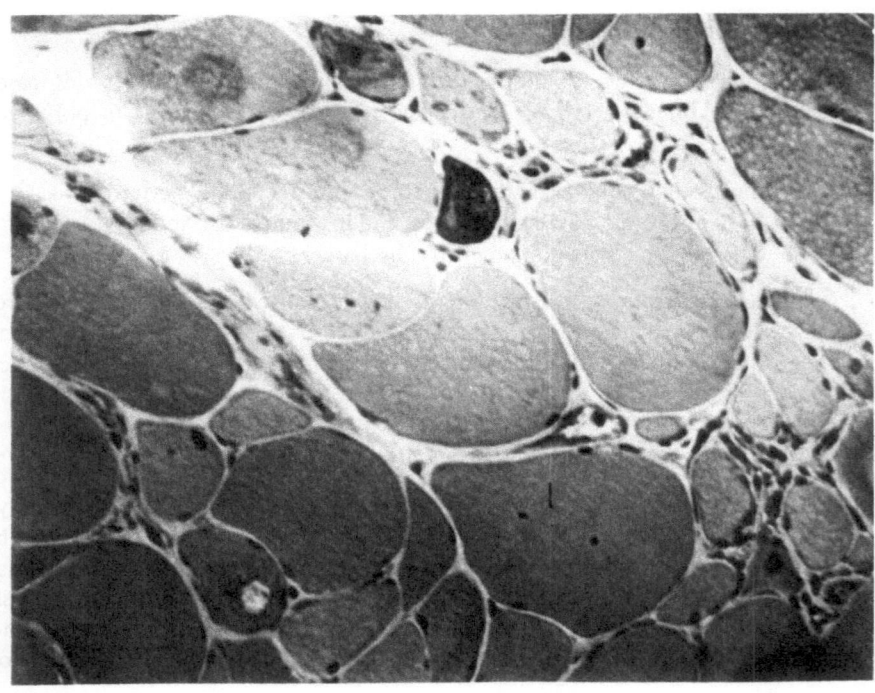

all of these changes are found in 80 to 90 percent of cases. Electron microscopic studies are of no additional value.

Other

Contrary to popular belief, the sedimentation rate (ESR) is not invariably elevated in polymyositis. DeVere and Bradley (1975) in their study of 118 patients with the disorder found an increased sedimentation rate in 55 percent of cases. Only 19 percent had a sedimentation rate above 50 mm./h.

Pathogenesis

The cause of polymyositis remains undetermined. Because of its common association with collagen vascular diseases and malignancies, it has long been suspected that the disease results from an altered immune state. To date, there is only sketchy evidence supporting a cellular and/or humeral mechanism in the disease. A viral etiology has been proposed by several investigators who have reported intranuclear and intracytoplasmic inclusions resembling viral particles in affected muscle tissue (Mastaglia et al, 1970). Further review of the pathogenesis of non-infections inflammatory muscle disease is provided by Whitaker (1982).

Prognosis and Treatment

Overall 70 percent of patients who are adequately treated improve. The prognosis for improvement is not in any way influenced by initial CPK values, EMG or biopsy findings. Improvement is greatest during the initial three years, and remains relatively constant thereafter. Most patients remain with a minimal degree of muscle weakness and wasting, and with little functional impairment. Patients who respond poorly to treatment are:

1. those who are either treated with inadequate doses of steroids, (less than 10 mg./day of prednisone) or whose treatment is delayed for more than one year;

2. those with polymyositis accompanying a well-defined collagen vascular disease particularly rheumatoid arthritis, systemic lupus erythematosus and progressive systemic sclerosis;

3. those who have a complicating malignant disease.

The overall mortality rate is between 15 and 25 percent and is highest in

---

Figure 8-4. Muscle biopsy—polymyositis. Note the extensive inflammatory infiltrate (A). Several fibers are seen undergoing active phagocytosis. (B) Note the fiber size variability and increased endomysial connective tissue which are nonspecific features of the myopathy.

those with an accompanying malignancy or collagen vascular disease. Polymyositis itself is rarely the casue of death in these patients with the majority of deaths resulting from other complications of their primary disease state, coronary artery disease, and pneumonia (Barwick and Walton, 1963; DeVere and Bradley, 1975).

High dose corticosteroids have been found to improve both mobidity and mortality. The recommended starting dose is 50 to 100 mg of prednisone daily, depending on the clinical severity of the disease. This dose is slowly readjusted to an alternate day schedule (i.e., 100 mg. Q.O.D.) (see Case 2, Chapter 3). Afterwards, reductions in the dose should be considered only after undertaking full monthly clinical and laboratory examinations (i.e., CPK) and assessing that the disease is in remission. Relapses occur in one-quarter of the cases and are usually the result of injudicious reductions in steroid dosage. Maintenance steroid doses probably should be continued for at least two years, although some believe that a shortened period of steroid therapy is more advisable in view of the well-known catabolic action of these drugs (Edwards, et al, 1979). If there is no response to steroids after six months of high dose prednisone, the patient should be given a trial of immunosuppressives. Those most widely used include cyclophosphamide (2 mg/kg/day) or azathioprine (3 mg/kg/day).

When immunosuppressives are given, one must warn the patient of the potential teratogenetic effects of these drugs. Pregnancy should be discouraged. With initiation of therapy, blood counts (i.e., hematocrit, hemoglobin, leukocytes, differential, and platelets) and tests of liver function (i.e., bilirubin, SGOT, SGPT, LDH, and alkaline phosphatase) should be done and repeated every two weeks during the initial six weeks of treatment. After this time, monthly blood studies will suffice. The therapeutic objective is to reduce the *lymphocyte* count to less than $1,000/mm^3$. Until this is achieved, there probably will be no response to the treatment. If the blood counts fall excessively (i.e., hematocrit under 30 percent, polymorphonuclear leukocytes under 800/ mm^3, or platelets under $50,000/mm^3$) or there is evidence of a chemical hepatitis, the drugs should be discontinued and restarted when the values return to normal.

An additional problem with azathioprine is its propensity to produce drug fevers. Fortunately, these fevers subside when the drug is stopped and usually do not reappear with reinstitution of therapy. Cyclophosphamide may produce a hemorrhagic cystitis and for this reason, patients taking the drug should be instructed to ingest large quantities of fluids daily.

Recently total body irradiation has been used successfully in a refractory case of polymyositis (Engel et al, 1981). However, such a procedure can only be carried out at neuromuscular centers under an approved research protocol.

Plasmapheresis in combination with immunosuppressive drug therapy can be used in patients whose disease is refractory to the more conventional modes of treatment (Dau 1981). However, the high cost of the procedure and the attending complications limit its use. All patients found to have myositis should be evaluated by a consulting oncologist. The vigor with which an occult malignancy screen is carried out, however, depends on the age and sex of the patient and whether there are accompanying skin manifestations (Figure 8-5).

Males over 40 years of age with dermatomyositis deserve the most complete search for an underlying malignancy. On the other hand, a child with dermatomyositis should be put through the rigors of an occult neoplasm screen unless there are specific symptoms and signs suggestive of a malignancy.

Case report

A 21-year-old woman consulted her physician because of weakness and muscle aches. For the past four months she noted difficulty washing and styling her hair, and complained that her arms felt heavy when held above her head. In addition, she had been avoiding the lower file cabinets at work because of difficulty rising from a squat. Muscle aches had become prominent in the past two months and seemed to be localized to the thighs. Physical examination revealed intact cranial nerve function but weakness in the shoulder and hip girdles. She complained of mild discomfort when the muscles of the proximal limbs were gently squeezed. Tendon reflexes were normal. Myositis seemed to be the most likely diagnosis but limb girdle dystrophy, endocrine myopathies, and adult-onset acid maltase deficiency, Eaton-Lambert syndrome and fasciitis were also considered. In order to clarify the problem, CPK, thyroid functions, and serum calcium and phosphate levels were ordered. Finding only a markedly elevated CPK (six times normal) a muscle biopsy was organized and appropriate stains were requested (see Table 2-1). The biopsy was compatible with inflammatory muscle disease and a limited occult malignancy evaluation was undertaken (i.e., chest x-ray, mammography, contrast study of the G. I. tract, and gynecologic evaluation). A neoplasm was not found and therapy was begun with prednisone 50 mg. daily. After three weeks, the patient's strength increased and her CPK fell to twice normal. However, because of unpleasant cosmetic side effects of the steroids (acne and hirsutism) she stopped the medication. Two weeks later, she had relapsed to her pre-treatment state. She was given azathioprine (3 mg/kg/day) and instructed about the hazards of becoming pregnant while on this medication. She returned for bimonthly examinations, blood counts and "liver function studies." She did well for three months but then developed unexplained fevers. Infectious disease evaluation was negative and it was felt that the fevers were drug induced. Azathioprine was discontinued and over the next 48 hours the fevers abated. She did well off all medications for two years but then relapsed. Treatment was reinstituted with cyclophosphamide (2 mg/kg/day). At the present time she is doing well and returns for monthly examinations and blood counts. Should she remain in remission, the cyclophosphamide will be discontinued in one year.

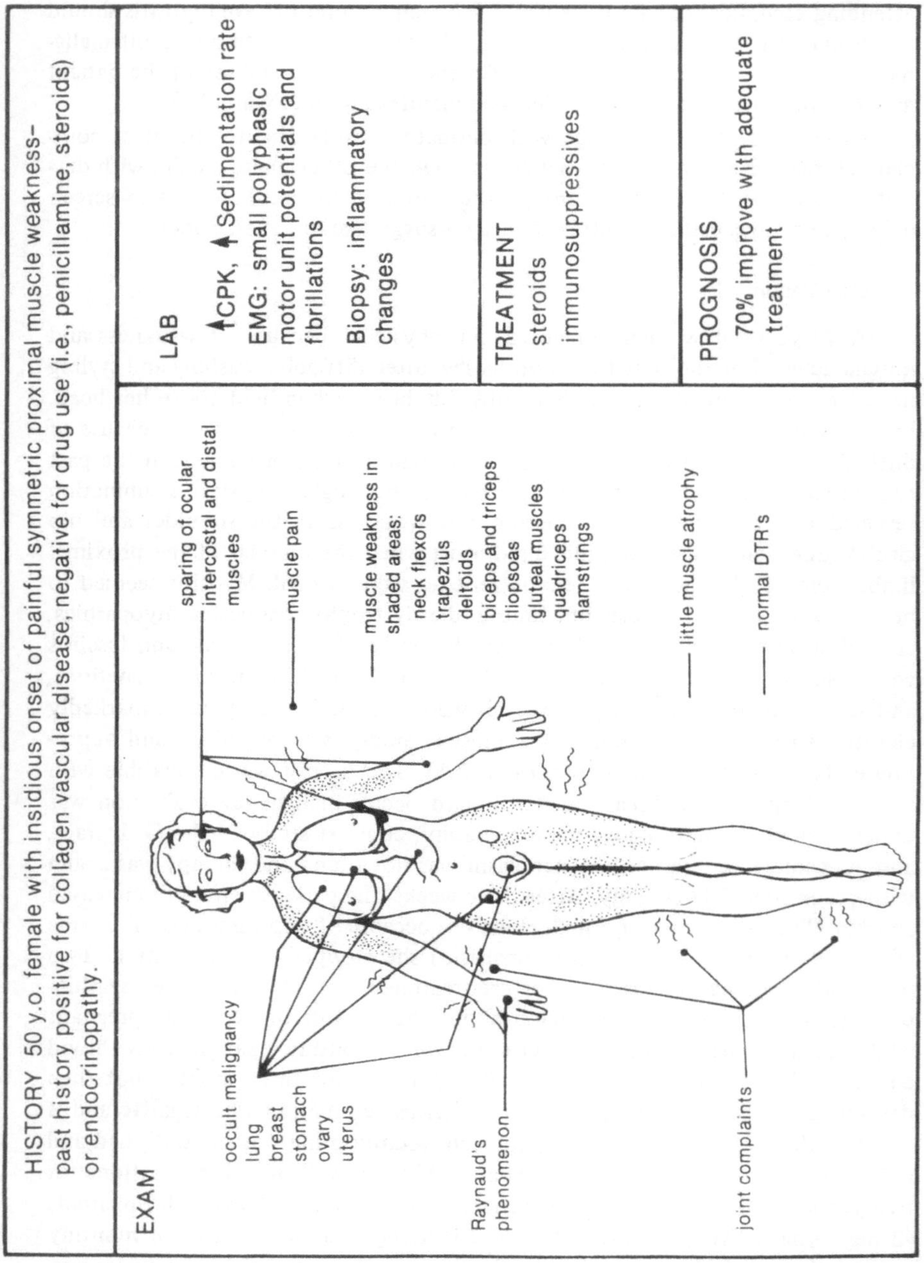

HISTORY 50 y.o. female with insidious onset of painful symmetric proximal muscle weakness—
past history positive for collagen vascular disease, negative for drug use (i.e., penicillamine, steroids)
or endocrinopathy.

EXAM

occult malignancy
lung
breast
stomach
ovary
uterus

Raynaud's
phenomenon

joint complaints

sparing of ocular
intercostal and distal
muscles

muscle pain

muscle weakness in
shaded areas:
neck flexors
trapezius
deltoids
biceps and triceps
iliopsoas
gluteal muscles
quadriceps
hamstrings

little muscle atrophy

normal DTR's

LAB

↑CPK, ↑ Sedimentation rate

EMG: small polyphasic
motor unit potentials and
fibrillations

Biopsy: inflammatory
changes

TREATMENT

steroids
immunosuppressives

PROGNOSIS

70% improve with adequate
treatment

Figure 8-5.   Summary of polymyositis.

CHILDHOOD DERMATOMYOSITIS

Childhood dermatomyositis (CD) is distinctive enough to be considered a specific entity. It differs from the adult variety in that the primary target of the disease process appears to be the blood vessels, and therefore the disorder is actually a systemic vasculopathy.

Onset of the disease is insidious with proximal lower extremity weakness being the earliest manifestation. As the disease progresses, proximal upper limb musculature as well as the muscles of deglutition weaken. Pain and tenderness of the involved muscles are common and the overlying skin may be indurated and edematous. Contractures frequently occur.

The skin lesions of CD are similar to those seen with the adult variety. Typically, there is violaceous discoloration of the upper lids and malar aspect of the face. Erythematous scaly lesions frequently cover the dorsi of the hands, elbows and knees. Calcinosis is a feature unique to CD. The calcification occurs in the interstitial tissues of the muscle and subcutaneous tissue. A calcium "paste" may be extruded through perforations in the skin.

Other organ systems are involved in the vasculopathy including the gastrointestinal (ulcerations) and genitourinary tracts. Pericarditis and arthralgias are frequent systemic manifestations as well.

There is no increased incidence of neoplasia with childhood dermatomyositis as there is in the adult variety.

Laboratory studies are sometimes needed to confirm the diagnosis and muscle biopsy is found to be the most helpful. Muscle tissue may at times show florid inflammatory changes but more commonly, the changes are minimal and may take the form of perifascicular atrophy. Thus, in view of the sparsity of inflammatory cells seen, it is not surprising that the sedimentation rate and serum CPK levels are normal in the majority of these patients. Electrodiagnostic studies reveal abundant polyphasic potentials for short duration and low amplitude (BSAPPs).

The course of the disease is variable with spontaneous remission in some cases. Most patients, however, experience a relapsing/remitting or chronically progressive course. Treatment is the same as in the adult variety.

INCLUSION BODY MYOSITIS

Inclusion body myositis (IBM) is a sporadic non-specific neuromuscular disease whose identification is based on morphologic studies. The initial case was reported by Chou (1967) who described a patient with slowly progressive weakness and a muscle biopsy showing intracytoplasmic vacuoles with tubular filaments. Additional cases have been subsequently reported and it now appears that these patients constitute a distinct clinopathologic entity called inclusion body myositis (see Danon et al, 1982 for a summary of cases reported to date).

Typically, cases of IBM present as progressive painless proximal muscle weakness. The biceps muscles may be disproportionately involved. Distal muscles are afflicted later in the course although in some instances, weakness of the hands is the presenting complaint. Such cases are frequently misdiagnosed as polyneuropathies or motor neuron disease. Myalgias are not prominent and bulbar musculature is generally spared. There are no skin manifestations or associated malignancies. Collagen-vascular diseases usually are not present except in one reported patient who also appeared to have Sjögren's syndrome (Chad et al, 1982). Unlike polymyositis, inclusion body myositis has an either normal or mildly elevated CPK and the disease does not respond to prednisone or immunosuppressive agents.

Diagnosis is confirmed .by muscle biopsy. Light microscopy reveals the typical changes ascribed to myopathies (i.e., fiber size variability, increased endomysial connective tissue, increased numbers of fibers with internal nuclei, and fibers undergoing degeneration and regeneration). In addition, there are mononuclear inflammatory infiltrates of varying degrees. The hallmarks of the disorder, however, are vacuoles lined with basophilic granules within muscle fibers. Some fibers have multiple vacuoles. These structures appear similar to the vacuoles described in patients with oculopharyngeal muscular dystrophy. Under the electron microscope the vacuoles are seen to contain abnormal filaments which may be viral products. However, viral isolation has been achieved in only one case of IBM (Mikol et al, 1982). These writers isolated an adenovirus type 2 from two successive muscle biopsy specimens taken from a patient with IBM. The question of whether or not the disease is caused by an atypical viral infestation of muscle remains to be answered.

In some cases the electrophysiologic and morphologic features are more in keeping with a neurogenic than a myopathic disorder (Eison et al, 1983).

FASCIITIS

Inflammation of investing fascial elements without involvement of the underlying muscle tissue may produce symptoms identical to polymyositis. Fasciitis may take several forms including eosinophilic fasciitis (EF), fascial inflammation associated with connective tissue disease, and fibrositis. An excellent discussion is provided by Simon et al (1982), and only a brief review will be presented here.

Eosinophilic fasciitis usually presents with pain in the extremities and trunk which is exacerbated by physical activity. Patients may complain of weakness but under examination, they have no real loss of muscle power. Instead, the skin and soft tissues overlying the painful muscles are found to be swollen and indurated. Limitation in the range of motion of the joints is also common. The disease afflicts men more often than women and the average age of onset is approximately forty years.

Laboratory studies are helpful in diagnosing the disorder. The vast majority of patients have increased numbers of circulating eosinophils which make up four to fifty percent of the total peripheral white count. Elevated sedimentation rate and gamma globulin levels are also generally found. In contrast to patients with polymyositis, trichinosis or other inflammatory myopathies, these patients have a normal CPK.

Definitive diagnosis can only be made by biopsy in which a piece of muscle fascia and underlying muscle are removed. With EF the fascia and fibrous septae between the muscle fascicles are thickened and infiltrated with mononuclear inflammatory cells and eosinophils. Muscle fiber necrosis and phagocytosis are generally not observed. Therefore, when evaluating a patient with muscle pain, and especially one with a normal CPK, a fascial biopsy and peripheral eosinophil count should be done. Otherwise the diagnosis of EF may be missed.

Treatment with prednisone (40-60 mg/day) is effective and results in prompt normalization of the sedimentation rate and eosinophilia. Clinical improvement occurs over months. If the patient does not respond to steroids, a trial of immunosuppressive drug therapy is indicated (azathiprine 3 mg/kg/day).

The collagen diseases including rheumatoid arthritis, systemic lupus erythematosus, scleroderma, polymyalgia rheumatica, Sjögren's syndrome and necrotizing vasculitides may be accompanied by a fasciitis. These diseases are unlike EF in that there are no peripheral eosinophilia or eosinophilic infiltrates in the muscle fascia.

Fibrositis is another disease included with the fascial inflammatory syndromes. This is an ill-defined entity characterized clinically by diffuse aches and pains. Discrete tender points are commonly discovered by these individuals. Biopsies are frequently normal. However, in some instances, lymphocytic infiltrates confined to the fascia are observed.

SARCOID MYOPATHY

Sarcoidosis is a common idiopathic granulomatous disease that may involve any organ system. Typically it is a chronic disorder, but may have acute stages characterized by fever, increased sedimentation rate, leukocytosis and myalgias. Central nervous system involvement is seen in approximately five percent of cases (Delaney, 1977). Such patients usually have other stigmata of the disease including skin changes, uveitis, parotitis, hilar adenopathy, anergy, hypercalcemia and a positive Kveim reaction. Central nervous system manifestations are generally secondary to a basal granulomatous meningitis with infiltration and compression of adjacent structures. Multiple cranial nerve palsies may result, with nerves VII, II, IX and X most frequently impaired. Hypothalamic and pituitary gland dysfunctions are also commonly a part of CNS sarcoidosis. Neuropathy that may take the form of polyneuropathy or mononeuritis multiplex is seen in 15 percent of cases.

Musculoskeletal involvement is much more common than was once believed; many patients with systemic sarcoidosis harbor a clinically silent myopathy. Approximately 60 percent of patients with systemic sarcoidosis but without muscle complaints or findings will have biopsy evidence of a granulomatous myopathy (Powell, 1953). On the other hand, symptomatic sarcoid myopathy, unlike CNS sarcoidosis may be the only clinical manifestation of the disease. In a recent review (Gardner-Thorpe, 1972), of 45 patients with clinically evident sarcoid myopathy, 40 percent had no other symptoms or signs of the disease at the time of diagnosis. However, isolated muscle sarcoidosis has never been confirmed by necropsy and it is doubtful that such an entity exists.

Clinical Presentation: Signs and Symptoms

Sarcoid myopathy, as previously discussed, may be asymptomatic or symptomatic. In the latter instance, painful palpable nodules overlying muscle may be the only clinical evidence of musculoskeletal involvement. More commonly, sarcoid myopathy manifests as weakness and atrophy in a distribution similar to that of the late-onset muscular dystrophies (Dyken, 1962). Such patients may have clinical evidence of systemic sarcoidosis and then the diagnosis is obvious. However, 40 to 60 percent do not manifest other signs and their clinical picture in the absence of a muscle biopsy is indistinguishable from that of muscular dystrophy, polymyositis, endocrine myopathy, adult acid maltase deficiency, muscle carnitine deficiency, or spinal muscular atrophy.

Typically, symptomatic sarcoid myopathy has its onset in the fifth to seventh decade. There is a 3:1 female preponderance. The predilection for postmenopausal women has led to speculation that there is a contributing endocrine factor, but as yet there is no proof of this. The myopathy affects the muscles of the proximal lower extremities most frequently, and a little less often, affects those of the shoulder girdle and proximal upper limbs. The patient initially complains of problems walking up stairs and is observed to have a waddling gait. Distal musculature may become involved but when it is prominent, one must consider a neurogenic cause. The muscle weakness and wasting is generally bilateral, symmetric, and does not include muscles of the face, eyes or neck. Pseudohypertrophy of the calves is occasionally seen and when present, may further confuse the clinical picture with that of a dystrophy. Cardiomyopathy frequently parallels skeletal muscle involvement. Muscle tenderness is rarely a major complaint. Diminished deep tendon reflexes and sensory abnormalities may be found when there is significant involvement of the peripheral nervous system.

Laboratory Studies

Serum muscle enzymes

Serum muscle enzyme determinations are of value. They are generally normal and, therefore may help to distinguish sarcoid myopathy from polymyositis.

Electromyography

Typical "myopathic" changes with EMG studies (i.e., small motor units) appear in about 75 percent of patients who have clinical evidence of muscle involvement. In approximately 10 to 20 percent of similar cases, both "myopathic" and neuropathic findings co-exist.

Muscle biopsy

The purpose of muscle biopsy in sarcoidosis is

1. to give a histological diagnosis in a suspected early case of the disease,
2. to confirm the etiology of muscle weakness in a known case of sarcoidosis.

When used to diagnose atypical cases of systemic sarcoidosis, routine sectioning of muscle at several levels is imperative becasue lesions are often sparsely situated in asymptotic individuals.

Characteristically, one observes spindle-shaped granulomata within and between the connective tissue sheaths of muscle fibers. Replacement of muscle fibers by fibrous and fatty tissue may also be seen. Occasionally, small granulomata coalesce to form large masses and produce clinically palpable nodules.

Pathogenesis

The pathogenesis of sarcoidosis is unknown. It seems that whether or not a given patient with the disease manifests musculoskeletal symptoms is directly related to the extent of granulomas in the muscle tissue. The granulomas when present compress and destroy adjacent muscle fibers, thus rendering them useless. Why some individuals with widespread systemic sarcoidosis have little muscle involvement while others have the opposite situation is unclear.

HISTORY   50 y.o. female with progressive painless lower extremity weakness, now involving the upper extremities. Past history positive for unexplained fevers, adenopathy and fatigue. Negative family history of muscle disease.

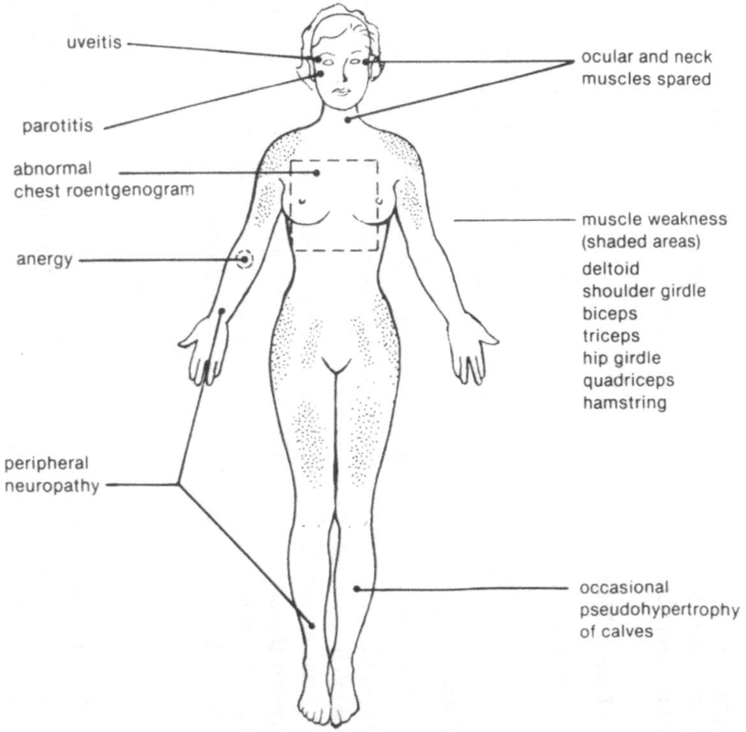

LAB

Normal CPK, ↑ Ca^{++}
CXR: hilar adenopathy
EMG: neuro-myopathic changes
Biopsy: granulomas in muscle tissue

TREATMENT

steroids

PROGNOSIS

uncertain

ocular and neck muscles spared

muscle weakness (shaded areas)

deltoid
shoulder girdle
biceps
triceps
hip girdle
quadriceps
hamstring

occasional pseudohypertrophy of calves

uveitis

parotitis

abnormal chest roentgenogram

anergy

peripheral neuropathy

Figure 8-6.   Summary of sarcoidosis.

Treatment and Course

Symptomatic sarcoid myopathy is a steadily progressive illness although fluctuations with exacerbations and remissions are common. Corticosteroids have been used to treat the myopathy but the response is at best unpredictable. In a series reported by Gardner-Thorpe (1972) 20 of the 26 patients with sarcoid myopathy improved on steroids. This improvement occurred over a two-month to a three-year period. The absence of other effective agents probably makes it advisable to use low dose steroids in patients with sarcoid myopathy. Figure 8-6 provides a summary of sarcoidosis.

CHAPTER 9

Disorders of Muscle Energy
Metabolism and Mitochondria

MUSCLE ENERGY METABOLISM

At the sub-cellular level skeletal muscle contraction involves the interaction and bonding of actin and myosin filaments (see Chapter 2). Energy is required for this process, and the phosphate bonds of adenosine triphosphate (ATP) provide the immediate source of this energy. Hydrolysis of the terminal phosphate bond of one mole of ATP liberates 7 to 8 kcal of energy.

$$ATP \longrightarrow ADP + Pi + 7\text{-}8 \, Kcal/mole$$

High energy phosphate bonds are stored in muscle in the form of phosphocreatine (PCr). This is readily converted to ATP.

$$PCr + ADP \xrightarrow[\text{phosphokinase}]{\text{creatine}} creatine + ATP$$

However, the amount of energy stored in this form is small and is rapidly depleted. Thus when a muscle is called upon to perform work, it must be capable of generating substantial amounts of ATP.

There are three principal substrates from which muscle tissue produces ATP. These include local muscle glycogen, serum glucose, and circulating free fatty acids. It seems that the particular fuel utilized is dependent upon several factors, most important of which are the duration and intensity of the work demanded and the immediate availability of a particular fuel. In addition, the state of oxygenation of the muscle tissue determines how the fuel substrate is ultimately metabolized.

159

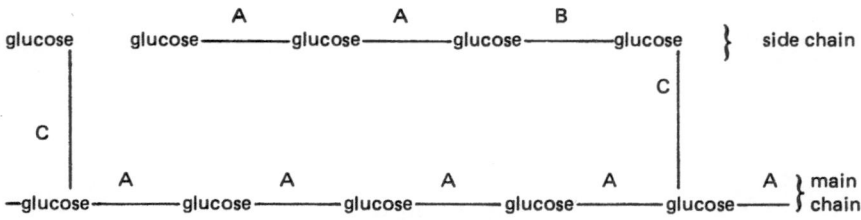

Glycogen

myophosphorylase: This enzyme phosphorylates α-1,4 glycosidic bonds (designated A) except those on the side chain immediately adjacent to the α-1,6 glycosidic bond. As a result, many glucose-1-phosphate units are produced.

oligo 1,4-1,4 glucantransferase: This enzyme cleaves the α-1,4 glycosidic bonds adjacent to the 1,6 bond on the side chain (designated B) and will add this unit to the main chain via an α1,4 bond.

amylo-1,6-glucosidase (debranching enzyme): This enzyme hydrolyzes the α-1,6 bond (designated C) to produce free glucose and a straight chain glycogen molecule.

Figure 9-1.   Glycogenolysis.

Within the cytoplasm of muscle fibers are found all the enzymes that catalyze the reactions of the Embden-Meyerhof pathway of anaerobic glycolysis. When short bursts of work of relatively high intensity are performed, local muscle glycogen serves as the main energy source. By the process of glycogenolysis (see Figure 9-1) glucose-1-phosphate molecules are produced. Glucose-1-phosphate after enzymatic conversion to glucose-6-phosphate is metabolized via the Embden-Meyerhof pathway with the subsequent generation of ATP, and lactate (see Figure 9-1). Approximately 3 to 4 moles of ATP per mole of glucose are produced by this chemical pathway.

At lower levels of sustained activity, muscle relies principally upon blood glucose (derived from hepatic glycogenolysis) and free fatty acids as its fuel substrates. Provided that there is adequate tissue oxygenation, pyruvate, the end product of glycolysis, is metabolized further to yield greater quantities of ATP. Muscle mitochondria are equipped with the enzymes and cofactors which constitute the Krebs cycle and cytochrome chain. Through these pathways, 36 to 39 moles of ATP are generated from 1 mole of glucose. (See Figures 9-3, 9-4 and 9-5.)

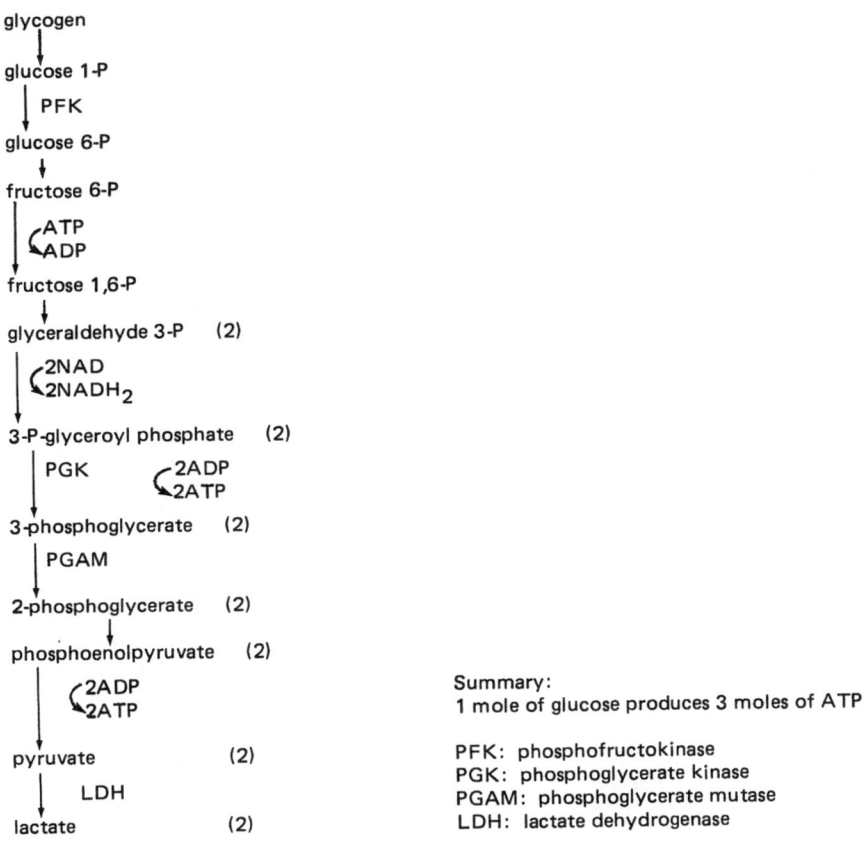

Figure 9-2.   Embden-Meyerhof pathway of anaerobic glycolysis.

Free fatty acids are derived from the hydrolysis of triglycerides stored in the body's adipose tissue. Fatty acids are oxidized within muscle mitochondria to multiple acetyl-CoA subunits. These molecules enter the Krebs cycle and ATP is thus generated (see Figure 9-6). To insure that adequate amounts of oxygen are available for aerobic metabolism, muscle tissue contains a unique oxygen binding protein called myoglobin. This molecule combines with oxygen and promotes its transport into the mitochondria where it serves as the terminal electron acceptor in the respiratory chain.

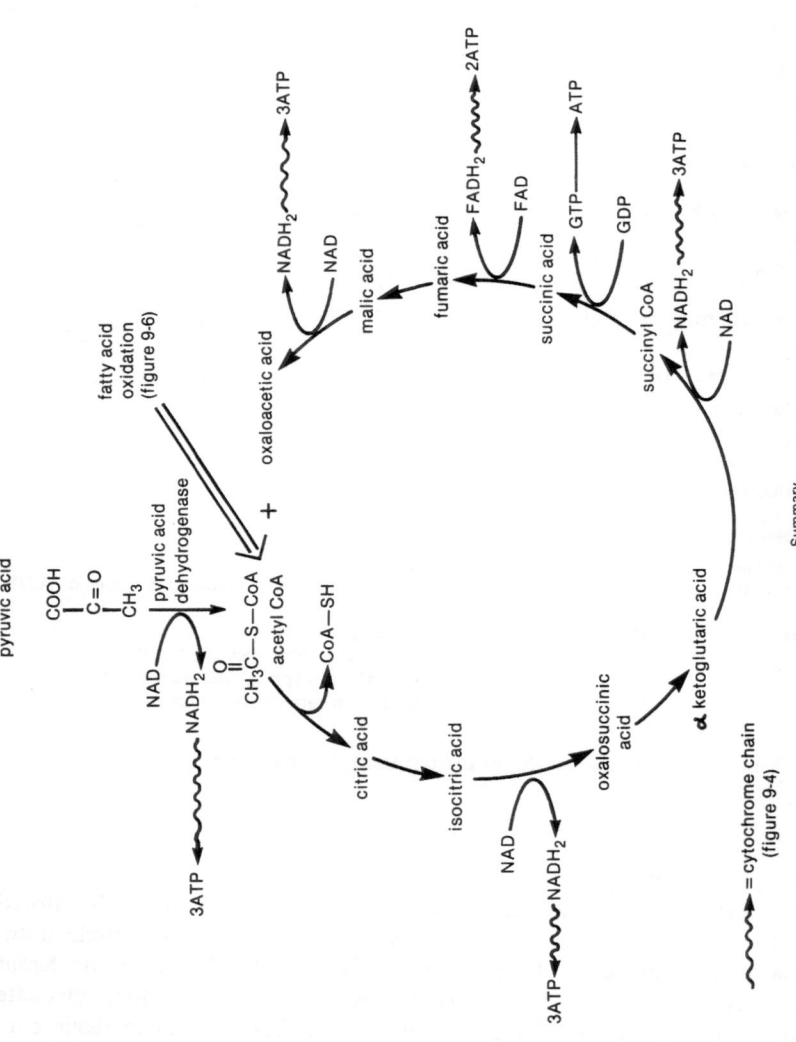

Figure 9-3. Krebs cycle.

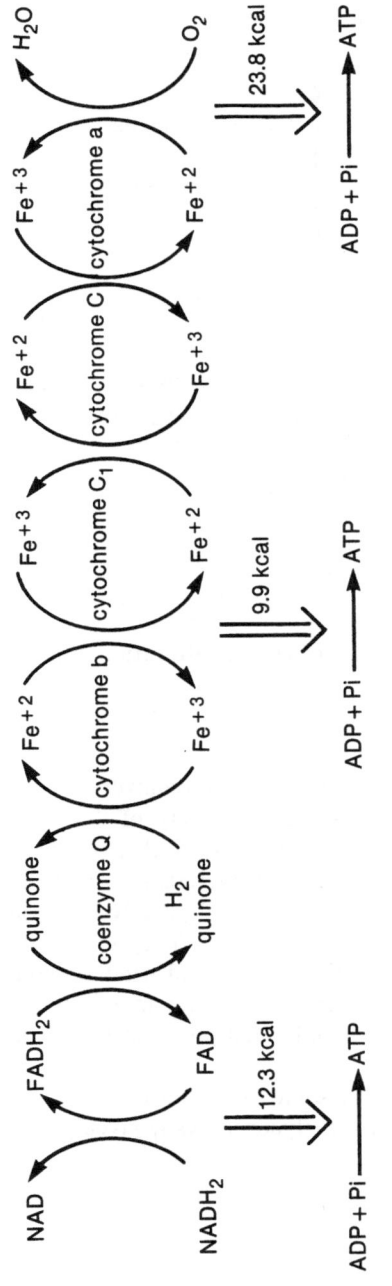

Summary

1 molecule of $NADH_2$ produces 3 molecules of ATP

Figure 9-4. Cytochrome chain.

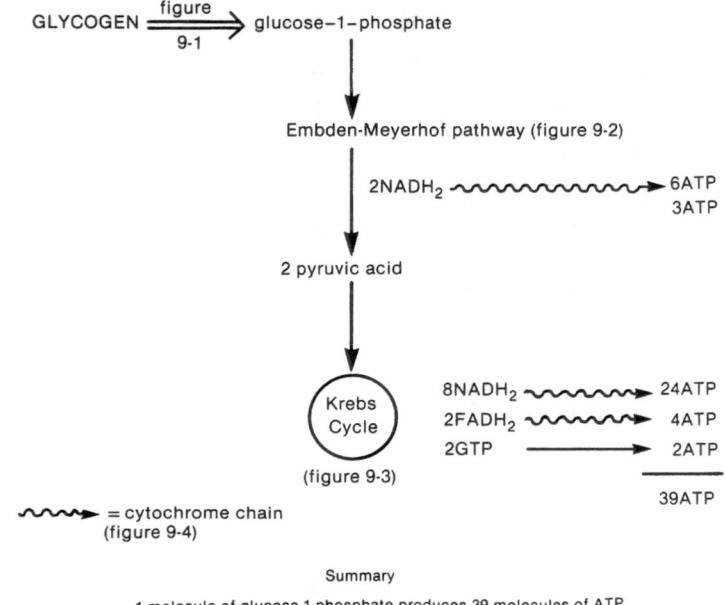

Summary

1 molecule of glucose-1-phosphate produces 39 molecules of ATP

Figure 9-5.   Summary of glucose utilization in muscle.

It is apparent that skeletal muscle tissue is omnivorous and utilizes a variety of fuels depending on the duration and intensity of the work that it is called upon to complete. Because of this need for fuel, patients with disorders of muscle energetics frequently manifest characteristic complaints. For example, patients with disorders of glycogenolysis and glycolysis become symptomatic when attempting short bursts of intense work. They may improve if they continue their activity at a lower level. This "second wind phenomenon" probably reflects their ability to mobilize and metabolize free fatty acids. In contrast, those afflicted with disorders of lipid transport usually become symptomatic after prolonged activity.

This chapter briefly describes some of the disorders of muscle metabolism. Included are disorders of myscle glycogenolysis, glycolysis fatty acid transport, and mitochondria.

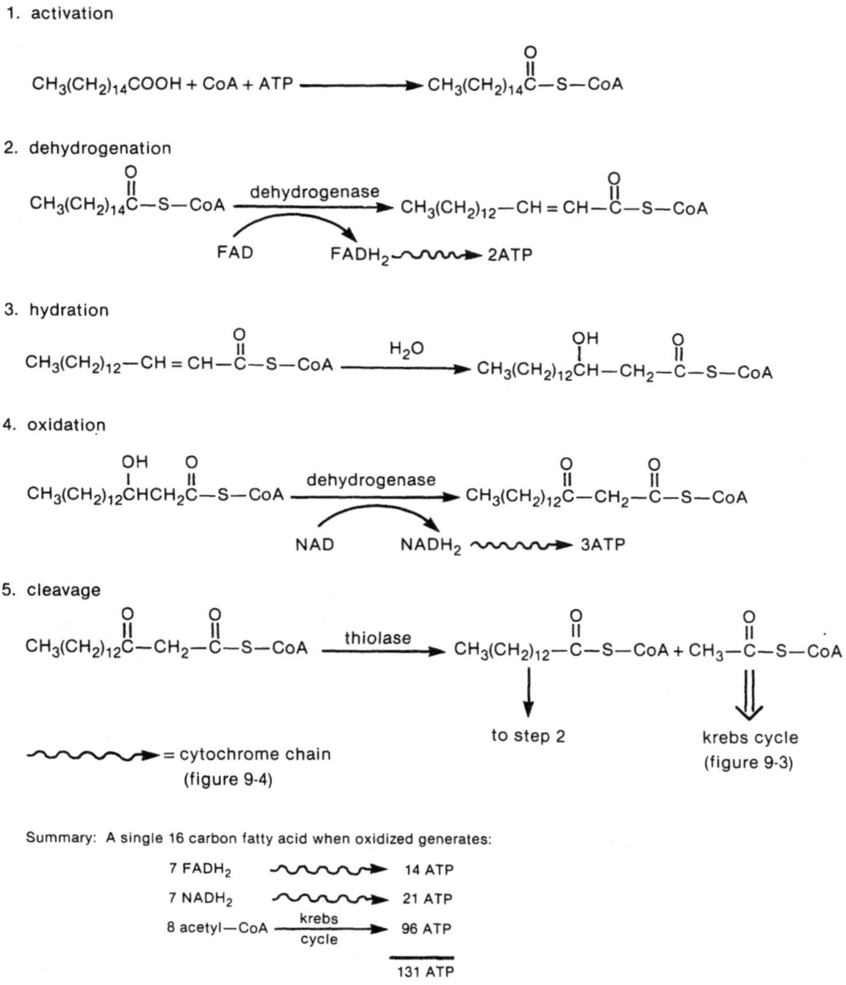

1. activation

$$CH_3(CH_2)_{14}COOH + CoA + ATP \longrightarrow CH_3(CH_2)_{14}\overset{O}{\overset{\|}{C}}-S-CoA$$

2. dehydrogenation

$$CH_3(CH_2)_{14}\overset{O}{\overset{\|}{C}}-S-CoA \xrightarrow[\text{dehydrogenase}]{} CH_3(CH_2)_{12}-CH=CH-\overset{O}{\overset{\|}{C}}-S-CoA$$

FAD   FADH$_2 \rightsquigarrow$ 2ATP

3. hydration

$$CH_3(CH_2)_{12}-CH=CH-\overset{O}{\overset{\|}{C}}-S-CoA \xrightarrow{H_2O} CH_3(CH_2)_{12}\overset{OH}{\overset{|}{C}H}-CH_2-\overset{O}{\overset{\|}{C}}-S-CoA$$

4. oxidation

$$CH_3(CH_2)_{12}\overset{OH}{\overset{|}{C}H}CH_2\overset{O}{\overset{\|}{C}}-S-CoA \xrightarrow[\text{dehydrogenase}]{} CH_3(CH_2)_{12}\overset{O}{\overset{\|}{C}}-CH_2-\overset{O}{\overset{\|}{C}}-S-CoA$$

NAD   NADH$_2 \rightsquigarrow$ 3ATP

5. cleavage

$$CH_3(CH_2)_{12}\overset{O}{\overset{\|}{C}}-CH_2-\overset{O}{\overset{\|}{C}}-S-CoA \xrightarrow{\text{thiolase}} CH_3(CH_2)_{12}-\overset{O}{\overset{\|}{C}}-S-CoA + CH_3-\overset{O}{\overset{\|}{C}}-S-CoA$$

$\rightsquigarrow$ = cytochrome chain
(figure 9-4)

to step 2   krebs cycle
(figure 9-3)

Summary: A single 16 carbon fatty acid when oxidized generates:

7 FADH$_2$ $\rightsquigarrow$ 14 ATP

7 NADH$_2$ $\rightsquigarrow$ 21 ATP

8 acetyl—CoA $\xrightarrow[\text{cycle}]{\text{krebs}}$ 96 ATP

_____
131 ATP

Figure 9-6. Oxidation of fatty acids [palmitic acid $CH_3(CH_2)_{14}COOH$].

Table 9-1.   Classification of the Glycogenoses

| | | | Tissues Affected | |
| | | | Skeletal Muscle | Other |
Type	Name	Deficient Enzyme		
I	von Gierke's	glucose-6-phosphatase	no	yes
II	Pompe's	acid maltase	yes	yes
III	Forbes', Cori's	amylo-1,6-glucosidase (debranching enzyme)	yes	yes
IV	Andersen's	amylo-1,4→1,6-transglucosidase (branching enzyme)	no	yes
V	McArdle's	myophosphorylase	yes	no
VI	Hers'	liver phosphorylase	no	yes
VII	Tarui's	phosphofructokinase	yes	no

THE GLYCOGENOSES

The glycogenoses are a group of disorders characterized by deranged glycogen and/or glucose metabolism. A numerical classification of these entities has been devised. However, there is some disagreement regarding this system (Table 9-1). Skeletal muscle is involved in five forms of the glycogenoses (Types II, III, IV, V and VII). In three of these (Types II, V and VII), muscle symptoms are the sole or predominant manifestation of the disease, whereas in types III and IV, symptoms of liver dysfunction and hypoglycemia dominate in clinical picture.

ACID MALTASE DEFICIENCY (TYPE II GLYCOGENOSIS)

Maltase (α-1,4-glucosidase) is an enzyme with widespread distribution whose specific function in carbohydrate metabolism is not clearly understood. It is a lysosomal enzyme which probably hydrolyzes glycogen to glucose, not as a necessity for energy supply, but as a scavenging mechanism of glycogen accidentally trapped in lysosomes after normal endocytosis. The absence of this enzyme is associated with accumulation of glycogen in lysosomes as well as free glycogen particles in the cell's cytoplasm.

Clinically, acid maltase deficiency (AMD) is a heterogenous disease. In the infantile form (Pompe's disease) enzymatic activity is absent in all tissues and glycogen accumulation is massive, especially in the skeletal muscles, heart, and central and peripheral nervous systems. Death from congestive heart failure before one year of age is common. In the late-onset variety, symptoms appear in adult life. The clinical picture is restricted to skeletal muscles and the disease may be confused with polymyositis or late-onset muscular dystrophy. The fact that there have been no families with both infantile and late-onset forms suggests that these are two distinct genetic disorders affecting the same enzyme.

Clinical Presentation: Signs and Symptoms

Both the infantile and adult-onset forms of acid maltase deficiency appear to be inherited in an autosomal recessive pattern. Newborns with the infantile variety appear normal at birth. However, within a few weeks, there is generalized hypotonia and weakness. Progressive hepatic enlargement and cardiomegaly secondary to glycogen accumulation are usually evident, and serve to distinguish these patients from those with spinal muscular atrophy (Werdnig-Hoffmann disease) and the other neuromuscular disorders which present as congenital hypotonia (see Figure 5-1). Macroglossia is occasionally seen. Death prior to age one from cardiorespiratory failure is inevitable.

In the late-onset variety of acid maltase deficiency, weakness develops in the third to fifth decades. There is no cardiac, visceral, or neuronal impairment. The weakness is slowly progressive and principally involves the muscles of the trunk and proximal limbs. Respiratory muscles are ultimately affected in over 50 percent of cases. Several patients have presented with respiratory failure as their initial manifestation (Rosenow and Engel, 1978). Adult-onset acid maltase deficiency may be confused with polymyositis, limb girdle muscular dystrophy, muscle carnitine deficiency and adult spinal muscular atrophies, all of which may present as proximal weakness without involvement of cranial musculature. Weakness of the respiratory muscles usually does not occur in these latter disorders and serves as a differentiating point. However, laboratory studies are needed to confirm the diagnosis of AMD.

Laboratory Studies

Serum muscle enzymes

Serum muscle enzyme levels are persistently but mildly elevated in both the infantile and adult-onset varieties of acid maltase deficiency. Asymptomatic heterozygotes may also have slightly increased serum concentrations of creatine phosphokinase and aldolase (Pellegrini et al, 1978).

Muscle biopsy

Typically, patients with acid maltase deficiency have vacuolar changes in their muscle tissue. These vacuoles contain PAS-positive material (glycogen) (see Figure 9-7).

At the ultrastructural level, glycogen particles are seen free in the cytoplasm

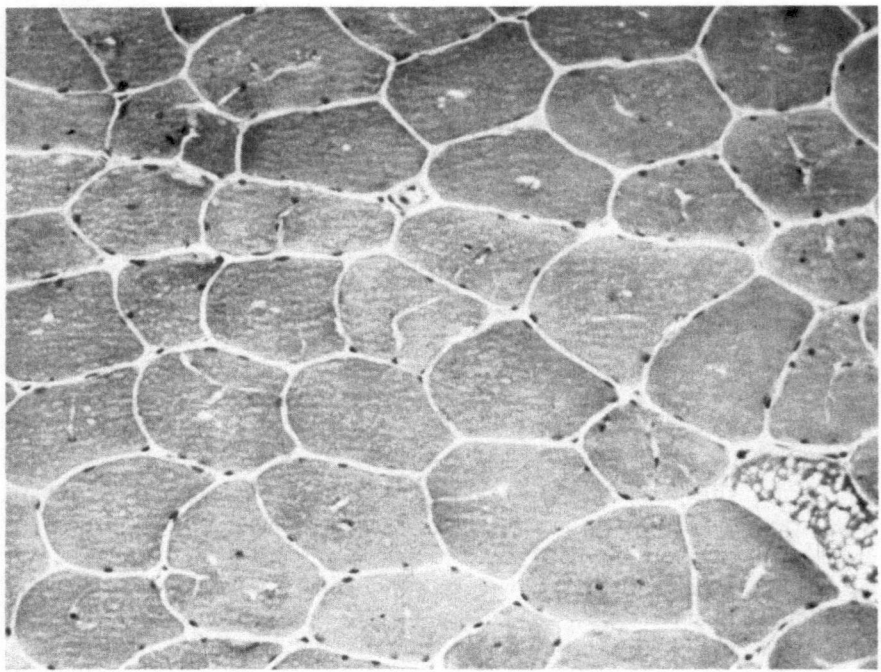

Figure 9-7. Muscle biopsy—acid maltase deficiency. Note the prominent vacuolar changes in the fiber at the lower right hand corner.

of muscle fibers as well as in membrane-bound vacuoles (Bertagnolio et al, 1978). Biochemical analysis of the muscle tissue reveals a complete absence of acid maltase activity in the infantile variety while in the adult form there is some residual enzyme activity.

Electromyography

Electrodiagnostic studies are particularly helpful in diagnosing the adult form of acid maltase deficiency. Myotonic discharges in the paraspinal muscles are characteristic of the disorder and may be the first clue that the patient does not have myositis or muscular dystrophy. In addition, brief, small, abundant polyphasic potentials (BSAPPs) are commonly seen in affected muscles.

Pathophysiology

Normally, cells form autophagic vacuoles which contain cellular particles isolated from the remainder of the cytoplasm by a membrane. These vacuoles merge with lysosomes to form autolysosomes. The components of the sequestered cytoplasm are digested by lysosomal enzymes, and some of the products pass through the membrane to be re-used by the cell while undigested material is retained or extruded. Absence of acid maltase, a lysosomal enzyme, prevents degradation of excess glycogen to glucose. The result is continued accumulation of undigested glycogen within lysosomes until the cell becomes engorged with these glycogenosomes. Such lysosomes may eventually break open and release destructive hydrolases intracellularly. Pressure atrophy may also play a role in the pathogenesis of the muscle weakness.

The biochemical basis of the clinical heterogeneity of acid maltase deficiency is uncertain. The fact that in the adult form there is some residual enzyme activity (between two and twelve percent of normal), while in the infantile variety the enzyme is totally absent, may explain the diverse clinical pictures (Mehler and Di Mauro, 1977; Di Mauro et al, 1978). Another belief is that in the adult variety, neutral maltase partially compensates for the low acid maltase levels (Angelini and Engel, 1972).

Treatment

Attempts have been made to treat the infantile variety with parenterally administered α-glucosidase. Both direct enzyme injections and enzyme administration via liposome carriers have been unsuccessful (Jacquemin et al, 1973).

Dietary manipulation has generally failed to alter the natural course of the disease. However, some have reported marked improvement in such patients when maintained on a high protein diet (Slonin et al, 1983).

Detection of heterozygotes is important for the purpose of genetic counselling. In the late-onset form, heterozygotes excrete approxmately 25 percent of the normal amount of acid maltase in the urine while those with the disorder (homozygotes) excrete about ten percent (Mehler and Di Mauro, 1977).

MYOPHOSPHORYLASE DEFICIENCY (McARDLE'S DISEASE: TYPE V GLYCOGENOSIS)

In 1951, McArdle described a 30-year-old patient with exertional muscle cramps and exercise intolerance. Serum lactate and pyruvate levels failed to rise after ischemic exercise. McArdle postulated a defect in carbohydrate metabolism. However it was not until eight years later, that the specific myophosphorylase enzyme deficiency was identified (Mommaerts et al, 1959; Schmid and Maher, 1959).

Phosphorylase is an enzyme normally found in a variety of tissues including liver and skeletal muscle. It is important for glycogenolysis (see Figure 9-1) and its absence prevents proper utilization of local glycogen stores for energy production.

In McArdle's disease, phosphorylase activity is normal in all tissues except skeletal muscle and for this reason, symptoms are restricted entirely to this system. Genetic, clinical, and biochemical evidence suggest at least three forms of this rare disorder: an autosomal dominant type which may have a more benign course (Chui and Munsat, 1976), and two autosomal recessive varieties—one in which there is a total absence of myophosphorylase biochemically and immunologically, and the other characterized by an altered enzyme protein, detectable immunologically but biochemically inactive (Feit and Brooke, 1976).

Clinical Presentation: Signs and Symptoms

Typically, McArdle's disease has three clinical stages. In childhood the disorder manifests itself as easy fatigability and reduced exercise tolerance. The second stage, which appears in early adult life, is dominated by muscle cramping and swelling and by the passage of darkly colored urine (myoglobinuria) after exercise. The degree of activity that may provoke such an episode varies from patient to patient. Some experience symptoms only after vigorous athletics while others have incapacitating muscle cramps and myoglobinuria following routine chores. Between attacks, patients appear normal and have no abnormalities on their physical examinations.

In the third stage of the illness, myoglobinuria is rare. However, the episodes of weakness and cramping are more easily provoked and last longer. At this time, permanent proximal muscle weakness may develop.

There are patients who do not follow the typical clinical pattern described above. A case of myophosphorylase deficiency presenting at birth with hypotonia and severe generalized weakness, and culminating in death at three months of age, has been reported (Di Mauro and Hartlage, 1978). In addition, Engel et al (1963) described a family in which the disease first appeared in the fifth decade. Generalized weakness without cramping or myoglobinuria characterized this family's variety of myophosphorylase deficiency.

The most common symptoms in subjects with McArdle's disease are an extremely low tolerance to physical activity, muscular fatigue, pain, and cramps. However, many find that if they are able to sustain exercise, these symptoms gradually disappear and they can continue. This improved performance has been called the second wind phenomenon and appears to result from the muscle's ability to mobilize and metabolize alternate fuels such as free fatty acids. In addition, increased muscle blood flow may contribute to the improved performance.

Except for possible renal failure, a life-threatening complication of myoglobinuria, McArdle's disease is, in general, an intermittent, relatively benign disorder. Between attacks, patients are normal and if they can avoid strenuous activity, they are able to enjoy nearly normal lives. Clinically, McArdle's disease is most apt to be confused with other disorders of energy metabolism (i.e., disorders of muscle glycolysis and lipid transport). Laboratory studies, including forearm ischemic exercise testing and muscle biopsy, are most helpful in differentiating these disorders.

Laboratory Studies

Serum muscle enzymes

Serum muscle enzyme levels may be elevated during an attack of muscle cramping and are invariably increased when myoglobinuria is present. In the interim between attacks, there are usualy no enzyme abnormalities.

Muscle biopsy

Muscle biopsy is the definitive method of diagnosing McArdle's disease. Absence of phosphorylase activity as demonstrated by histochemical techniques is the hallmark of the disorder. In addition, muscle fibers with subsarcolemmal blebs containing glycogen may be seen in the disease (Dubowitz and Brooke, 1973) (see Figure 9-8). If the biopsy is done after vigorous exercise, abundant necrotic fibers may be apparent.

Electromyography

Insertion of concentric needle electrodes in the forearm flexor muscles following ischemic exercise demonstrates that the contractured muscle is electrically silent. Electrical testing prior to an attack is usually normal. However, if the disease is longstanding, a "BSAPP" pattern may appear.

Ischemic exercise test

The ischemic exercise test is a rapid and easy screening test for disorders of glycogenolysis and glycolysis (see Figure 9-9). Work performed under ischemic conditions normally produces a two- to five-fold rise in serum lactate levels. Patients with McArdle's disease are unable to utilize local glycogen stores, and therefore do not produce lactate or pyruvate when deprived of blood derived fuel substrates. With disorders of muscle glycolysis there will also be an abnormal ischemic exercise test. However, the muscle biopsy will confirm the presence of myophosphorylase activity in these patients.

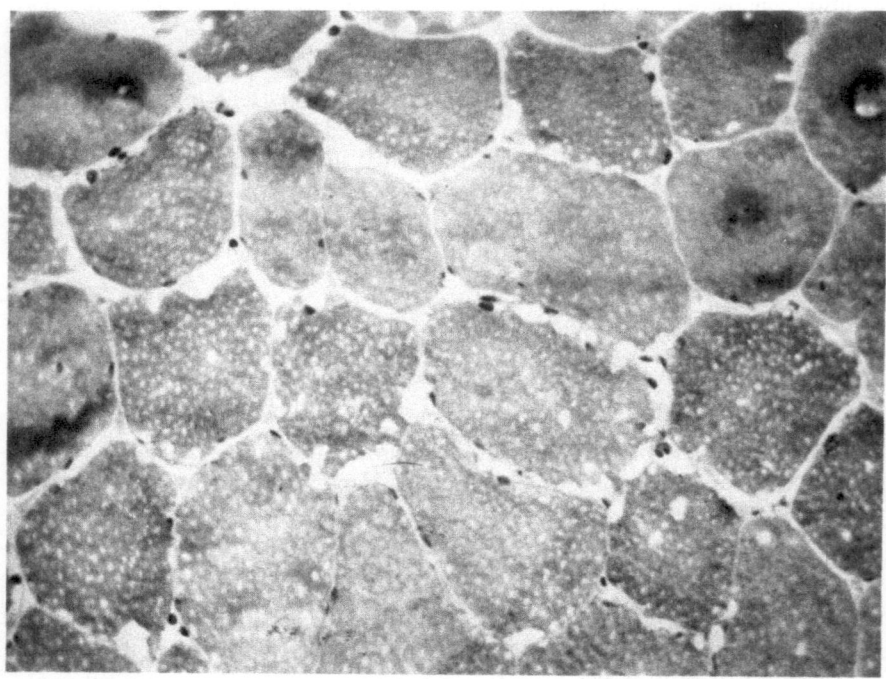

Figure 9-8. Muscle biopsy—myophosphorylase deficiency. Note the abundant large subsarcolemmal vacuoles. (The smaller, more numerous vacuoles are freeze artifact.)

A new non-invasive technique using phosphorous nuclear magnetic resonance can be used to measure intramuscular pH and high energy phosphate compounds (Ross et al, 1981). Working under ischemic conditions, normal muscle becomes acidotic and eventually depletes its stores of creatine phosphate. Under similar conditions, muscle of patients with McArdle's disease will show a much smaller decline in pH but a much accelerated depletion of creatine phosphate. This non-invasive technique of monitoring muscle metabolism under ischemic conditions can be used to test various therapies in patients with McArdle's syndrome.

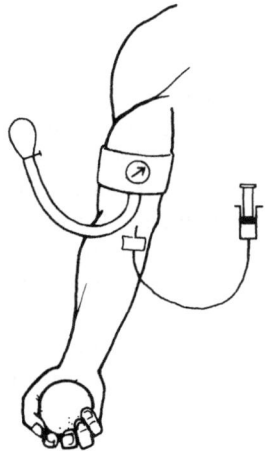

1. Insert heparin lock.
2. Draw venous blood at rest for lactate (time 0).
3. Inflate blood pressure cuff on upper arm to above systolic blood pressure.
4. Exercise hand and forearm muscles to fatigue (i.e., squeeze sponge ball).
5. Draw venous blood for lactate immediately after exercise and at 1, 2, 4, 6 and 10 minutes after fatigue point is reached.

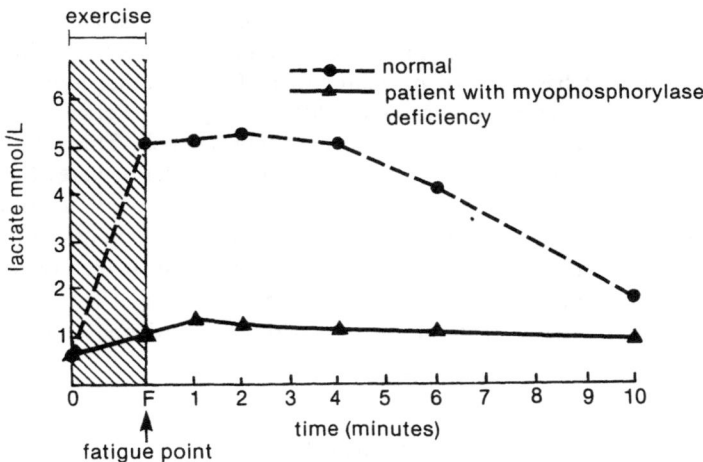

Figure 9-9. Ischemic exercise test.

Pathophysiology

McArdle's disease is the first of the hereditary myopathies in which the metabolic defect was elucidated. The absence of phosphorylase activity with subsequent impaired glycogen utilization and energy production accounts for the muscle cramping and weakness, and myoglobinuria with exertion.

During rest or light work, muscle is capable of supplying its energy needs entirely from the oxidative metabolism of fatty acids and glucose. During vigorous work, this souce is insufficient for one or more reasons: the relative isechemia of contracting muscles; the relative slowness of oxidative metabolism; and limitations in the rate of entry of substrates such as fatty acids. Thus local glycogen is the major fuel source for short bursts of activity. With myophosphorylase deficiency, muscle glycogenolysis is impossible and vigorous exercise precipitates bouts of muscle necrosis.

Treatment

Patients with myophosphorylase deficiency must avoid "strenuous" physical activity. For some patients, this involves minor adjustments in life style such as playing first base instead of center field. But for other more severely afflicted individuals, over-exertion can mean lifting a bag of groceries.

Treatment is aimed at bypassing the biochemical block. This may be accomplished by supplying the muscles with glycolytic intermediates (i.e., glucose, fructose) or with free fatty acids (Rowland et al, 1963). Patients should be instructed to ingest high glucose-containing foods (i.e., honey, molasses, glucose drinks) prior to anticipated muscular exertion. Such dietary management does seem to improve exercise performance. However, it is inconvenient and results in substantial weight gain in the majority of patients. An illustrative case history follows.

Case Report

An 11 year-old boy was brought to a psychiatrist because of suspected hypochondriasis. For two years he had complained of work related fatigue and muscle aches. His father, growing more intolerant of his son's apparent laziness, frequently punished him for not completing his chores. Unable to find evidence of a personality disorder, the psychiatrist suggested that the boy see a pediatrician, but this request went ignored. Two years later, the boy was brought to the pediatrician's office with severe diffuse muscle cramps. That afternoon the boy was told to chop firewood but after several minutes stopped because of pain in his hands and shoulders. He was ordered to continue by his enranged father and minutes later collapsed in pain. He was unable to release the axe handle from his cramped hands. In the pediatrician's office, the boy voided a large amount of tea-colored urine. Suspecting a metabolic myopathy the physician had the urine analyzed for myoglobin (which was present) and the boy was hospitalized. On admission, his CPK was found to be six times normal. He was kept well hydrated with 7 liters of daily intravenous fluids and the pain was treated with mild analgesics. After three days he felt well. An ischemic exercise test was done and during this procedure there was no increase in the serum lactate or pyruvate levels. To further clarify the situation, a muscle biopsy was arranged. Myophosphorylase and oil red O stains were specifically requested. The diagnosis of McArdle's disease was confirmed by the absence of myophosphorylase activity in the muscle tissue. The boy was referred to a neuromuscular disease center for further investigation and treatment.

PHOSPHOFRUCTOKINASE DEFICIENCY (TARUI'S DISEASE: TYPE VII GLYCOGENOSIS)

In 1965 Tarui et al described a rare familial muscle disorder whose clinical characteristics closely mimicked those of McArdle's disease. Afflicted individuals complained of easy fatigability, muscle cramping, and stiffness when subjected to vigorous exercise. Unlike those with McArdle's disease, these patients had normal myophosphorylase activity but absent phosphofructokinase (PFK). Becasue of this enzymatic deficiency, glycogen accumulated in the muscle fibers and this disorder was added to the list of glycogenoses.

Biochemical studies subsequently have shown that affected patients have absent PFK activity in muscle and a 50 percent reduction in erythrocytes (Layzer et al, 1967; Tarui et al, 1969). Apparently, erythrocyte PFK is composed of two distinct subunits, designated M and R, whereas muscle PFK contains only M subunits. These two subunits are under different genetic control and Tarui's disease results from a deficiency of M subunits. Consequently, patients with the disorder may manifest features of mild hemolytic disease (reduced red blood cell life span, erythroid hyperplasia of the bone marrow, and increased reticulocyte counts) in addition to neuromuscular symptoms (Tarui et al, 1969).

Clinical Presentation: Signs and Symptoms

Patients with PFK deficiency suffer from early childhood with exercise intolerance and painful muscle cramps, often accompanied by nausea and myoglobinuria. Just like patients with McArdle's disease, they often find that if they are able to sustain activity when cramping develops, the symptoms may subside. This second wind phenomenon may reflect the muscle's ability to utilize substrates other than glucose.

At rest, patients with PFK deficiency are normal and by limiting exertion, such individuals are able to lead relatively normal lives.

Laboratory Studies

Serum muscle enzymes

After exertion, serum muscle enzymes may be elevated and myoglobinuria may be evident.

Muscle biopsy

Muscle biopsy is essential to distinguish these patients from those with McArdle's disease. Under the light microscope, both disorders show similar pathologic changes including increased muscle glycogen, and muscle fibers with subsarcolemmal vacuoles. However, histochemical staining for phosphorylase is absent in McArdle's disease but present in PFK deficiency. The definitive diagnosis is made by demonstrating an absence of PFK activity in the muscle tissue. Patients with the disorder are found to have only two to six percent of normal PFK activity. A histochemical technique to demonstrate PFK activity has been described (Bonilla and Schotland, 1970).

Ischemic exercise test

As with patients with myophosphorylase deficiency, patients with Tarui's disease do not produce lactate or pyruvate when they exercise under ischemic conditions (see Figure 9-9).

Painful contractures of forearm muscles appear during ischemic exercise and result in involuntary flexion of the wrist and fingers. It may take several hours for this condition to abate.

Pathophysiology

Phosphofructokinase catalyzes the conversion of fructose-6-phosphate to fructose-1,6-diphosphate (see Figure 9-2). This enzymatic step is one of the main rate-limiting steps of glycolysis. The block in the Embden-Meyerhof pathway occurs prior to those steps which produce ATP. Therefore ATP cannot be generated from either glycogen or glucose.

The site of the enzyme deficiency has been verified by demonstrating that muscle homogenates from patients with the disorder produce lactate and pyruvate when supplied with substrates beyond the PFK step in glycolysis.

Treatment

Because the metabolic block affects glycolysis rather than glycogenolysis there is no rationale for the administration of glucose of hyperglycemic agents. Dietary supplementation with ketone bodies or fatty acids (Portagen) may be of benefit (Di Mauro and Eastwood, 1977).

OTHER DISORDERS OF MUSCLE GLUCOSE METABOLISM

Recently three new enzyme defects of muscle glycolysis have been identified. The enzymes involved in these disorders are phosphoglycerate kinase (PGK) (Di Mauro et al, 1982), phosphoglycerate mutase (PGAM) (Di Mauro et al, 1982; Bresolin et al, 1983), and lactate dehydrogenase (LDH) (Kanno et al, 1980). All three disorders are characterized by exercise-induced muscle cramps (but no fixed weakness), and recurrent myoglobinuria. Because the enzymatic "block" occurs in the steps preceding lactate formation (see Figure 9-2) the ischemic exercise test will be abnormal in all three. Only muscle biopsy and measurement of individual glycolytic enzymes can differentiate these entities from myophosphorylase and PFK deficiency.

FATTY ACID TRANSPORT

Lipids are at least as important as glycogen as a source of energy for muscle contraction. Glycogen breakdown is suited for rapid provison of energy during strenuous effort but muscle glycogenolysis cannot sustain exercise for more than a few minutes. The energy for prolonged efforts derives mainly from lipids. Circulating fatty acids enter the muscle fiber and are activated at the surface of the outer mitochondrial membrane at the expense of ATP. The acyl-CoA formed is then transferred from coenzyme A to carnitine by carnitine palmityl transferase I (CPT I) located on the outer aspect of the inner mitochondrial membrane.

Carnitine is the obligatory carrier of long chain fatty acids through the inner mitochondrial barrier to the site of B-oxidation and ketone production. It is synthesized in the liver and reaches other tissues via the circulation. As the carnitine level in skeletal and cardiac muscle greatly exceeds that in the serum, it is believed that carnitine uptake by these tissues depends on an active transport mechanism (Willner et al, 1978). If carnitine is lacking, muscle fatty acid metabolism is severely impaired (Long et al, 1982) and the acyl-CoA is converted to triacylglycerol of fat droplets.

On the inner aspect of the inner mitochondrial membrane, a second carni-

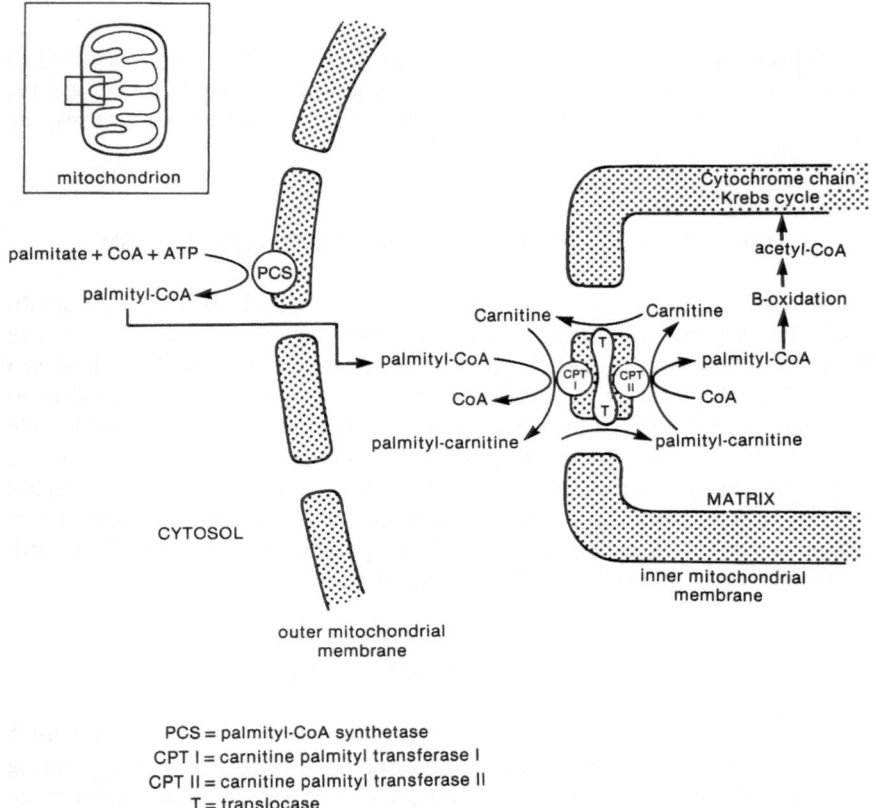

PCS = palmityl-CoA synthetase
CPT I = carnitine palmityl transferase I
CPT II = carnitine palmityl transferase II
    T = translocase

Figure 9-10. Fatty acid transport into mitochondria.

palmity transferase (CPT II) catalyzes the reverse reaction, reconverting fatty acyl-carnitine to fatty acyl-CoA (see Figure 9-10). Beta-oxidation of fatty acyl-CoA within mitochondria (see Figure 9-6) generates multiple acetyl-CoA subunits which then enter the Krebs cycle for ATP production (see Figure 9-3).

It is of note that the inner mitochondrial membrane is impermeable to carnitine and acylcarnitine as it is to CoA and its esters. A translocase system, however, operates to exchange free carnitine and acylcarnitine at this site (Pande, 1975). To date several disorders of muscle lipid metabolism have been described. One is characterized by progressive weakness (carnitine deficiency) while in the other, episodic muscle pain and myoglobinuria prevail (carnitine palmityl transferase deficiency). There are many reported patients with lipid storage myopathy in whom neither carnitine nor CPT is deficient. In these cases, the precise biochemical error remains to be identified (Di Mauro et al, 1980).

CARNITINE DEFICIENCY

Two varieties of human carnitine deficiency have been described to date. In the systemic form of the disease, hepatic, serum and extra-hepatic tissue concentrations of carnitine are diminished. Intermittent episodes of hepatomegaly, liver dysfunction, and acidosis, which may be fatal, characterize the disorder. Myopathy usually develops later in the illness. In the second type of carnitine deficiency, carnitine levels are normal in the liver and plasma but are markedly decreased in muscle tissue. Patients suffering from muscle carnitine deficiency manifest muscle weakness but do not experience bouts of liver dysfunction, acidosis, or encephalopathy. Although a few patients share characteristics of both forms, this subdivision distinguishes two reasonably homogenous groups of patients. It is believed that both varieties are inherited in an autosomal recessive pattern.

The fact that an increasing number of patients have been diagnosed as suffering from carnitine deficiency since the initial description of the syndrome in 1972 (Engel and Siekert, 1972; Engel and Angelini, 1973) suggests that the disease is not uncommon. While not all cases of lipid storage myopathy are due to carnitine deficiency, recognition of the disease by appropriate histological and biochemical tests is important because it is a potentially fatal, yet treatable illness.

Clinical Presentation: Signs and Symptoms

The clinical picture of systemic carnitine deficiency is variable. In most patients, a pre-myopathic phase lasting two to ten years antedates the development of muscle weakness. In some patients, episodes of nonketonic hypoglycemia without encephalopathy may precede the encephalopathic phase (Slonim et al, 1983). Other patients experience recurrent bouts of profound asthenia, adynamia, anorexia, nausea, vomiting, and mental confusion reminiscent of Reye's syndrome. Fasting may be a precipitating factor although most episodes occur spontaneously. These paroxysms may have their onset in infancy, early childhood, or adolescence. During these episodes, there is hepatomegaly and biochemical evidence of liver dysfunction with or without renal failure (Karpati et al, 1975; Cornelio et al, 1977). Elevated liver enzymes, acidosis, and uremia may be prominent findings. With supportive care, the metabolic encephalopathy and acidosis generally abate within days or weeks. However, patients have died from irreversible liver and renal dysfunction (Engel et al, 1977). In most cases, a proximal myopathy appears subsequently which may be aggravated by pregnancy or be accelerated during the episodes of acidosis and encephalopathy. Systemic carnitine deficiency should be suspected in all children with unexplained mild or severe myopathy and evidence of impaired liver function.

In contrast, patients with muscle carnitine deficiency present at a variable age (usually childhood) with proximal muscle weakness. A fatal cardiomyopathy may occasionally be part of the clinical picture (Hart et al, 1978). Because bulbar muscles are seldom involved and liver dysfunction does not occur, the disease can be easily mistaken for one of the dystrophies or spinal muscular atrophies. Since these latter disorders are untreatable, it would be tragic to assume such diagnosis without further investigative studies to rule out correctable conditions such as muscle carnitine deficiency.

Laboratory Studies

Blood studies

As previously mentioned, biochemical evidence of liver and renal dysfunction may be present during the encephalopathic episodes of systemic carnitine deficiency. In addition, the serum creatine phosphokinase (CPK) may be elevated and there is usually an accompanying metabolic acidosis. Patients with carnitine deficiency restricted to the muscles have mildly elevated CPK levels without biochemical evidence of hepatic or renal insufficiency.

Muscle biopsy

Biopsy of skeletal muscles in both varieties of the disease reveal muscle fibers with abundant slit-like spaces. These changes are more prominent in type I fibers. Staining with oil red O demonstrates that the spaces contain neutral lipids (see Figure 9-11). Electron microscopic studies of biopsy specimens frequently reveal increased numbers of mitochondria which are morphologically abnormal (Karpati et al, 1975).

Electrodiagnostic tests

Typically, electromyographic studies show a "BSAPP" pattern in affected muscles. However, in one case, there were reduced conduction velocities indicating neuronal (Schwann cell) involvement (Markesbery et al, 1974).

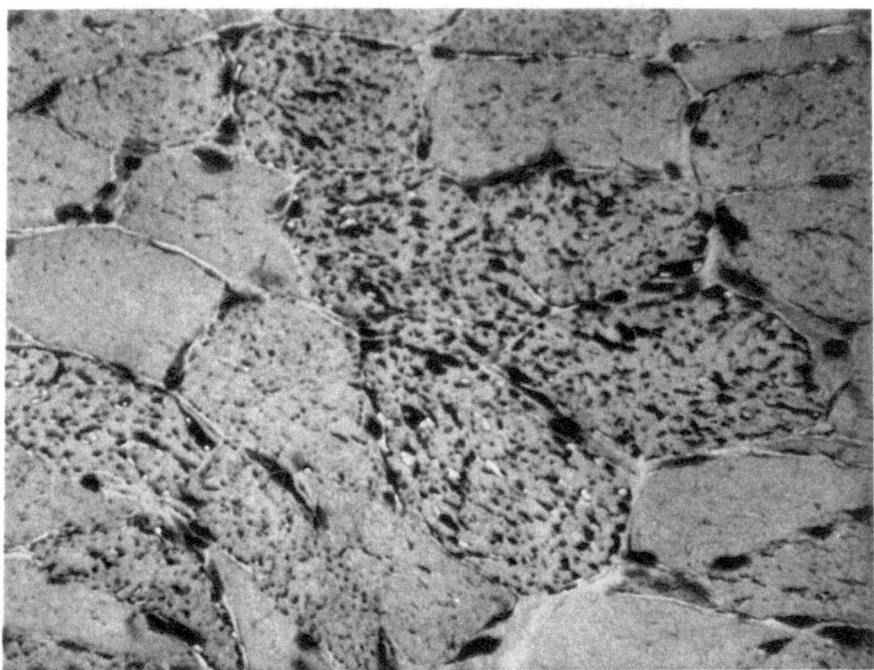

Figure 9-11. Muscle biopsy—carnitine deficiency (Oil Red O Stain). Note the excessive amount of lipid (dark staining material) in many fibers.

Other

Patients with muscle carnitine deficiency have low levels of carnitine only in skeletal and cardiac muscle. Those with the systemic variety have reduced levels in the liver and serum as well as in the muscles. Normal values for free and total carnitine in serum, skeletal muscle, and liver are listed in Table 9-2. Measuring serum ketones, lactate and pyruvate levels after fasting may be helpful in differentiating the muscle form from the systemic variety of carnitine deficiency. In the type restricted to the skeletal muscles, fasting is accompanied by a profound ketonemia, reflecting an exaggerated response of the intact liver to caloric deprivation. In the systemic form, plasma ketones rise very little with fasting but instead there are elevated levels of lactate and pyruvate. This latter phenomenon is probably a consequence of enhanced muscle glycolysis (Di Donato et al, 1980). Because fasting may initiate a series of catastrophic

Table 9-2. Normal Values of Carnitine in Serum (or Plasma)
and Tissues (Rebouche and Engel, 1983)

	Free Carnitine	Total Carnitine
	Serum (plasma) (nmol/ml)	
mean ± SD (males)	46.8 ± 10.0	59.3 ± 11.9
mean ± SD (females)	40.1 ± 9.5	51.5 ± 11.6
	Skeletal muscle (nmol/mg NCP)	
mean ± SD (males)	18.0 ± 8.1	20.5 ± 8.4
mean ± SD (females)	17.3 ± 5.3	20.1 ± 5.3
	Liver (nmol/mg NCP)	
mean	7.3	10.2

NCP - non-collagen protein.

catastrophic events in patients with systemic carnitine deficiency, such testing
should be done with extreme caution.

Pathophysiology

Impaired synthesis of carnitine is the postulated but not proven underlying
defect in systemic carnitine deficiency. In support of this theory is the report
of Slonim and associates (1983) who found decreased γ-butyrobetaine hydroxy-
lase activity in a single case of SCD. (This is the enzyme involved in the last step
of carnitine biosynthesis.) However, in other patients with SCD, synthesis appears to be normal. In SCD, both liver and muscle mitochondria are unable to
transport long chain fatty acids into the interior matrix for beta-oxidation and
ATP production. Instead, fatty acids are converted to neutral fat droplets which
accumulate in tissues including the liver and skeletal muscle fibers. The liver
compensates for the carnitine deficiency by increasing omega-oxidation of fatty
acids. This is an extra-mitochondrial process which results in high serum levels
of dicarboxylic acids. These acids are readily detected in the urine of such patients and are in part responsible for the systemic acidosis (Engel et al, 1977).

Accumulation of excessive fatty acids in hepatocytes eventually leads to
hepatomegaly, generalized liver insufficiency, and encephalopathy. Muscle
weakness occurs as a consequence of impaired B-oxidation of fatty acids and
diminished ATP production.

In muscle carnitine deficiency, the normal serum and liver carnitine concentrations suggest that synthesis is not impaired. A defect in transport of
carnitine from the plasma into muscle fibers is the most likely cause of the
syndrome. Because liver metabolism is not impaired, acidosis, hypoglycemia,
and encephalopathy do not occur. Ketone production is generally normal.

Treatment

Because fasting may produce a fatal acidosis, patients with systemic carnitine deficiency should be warned about skipping meals or injudicious dieting. Supplementing the diet of such patients with MCT oil is helpful since oxidation of these medium chain lipids does not require the carnitine carrier. Oral carnitine should be given in all cases of carnitine deficiency. Doses of 1.5 to 18 g/day of D,L-carnitine have produced improvement in a number of cases (Angelini et al, 1976; Hosking et al, 1977). Carnitine is relatively free of toxic side effects. Nausea and diarrhea may be noted initially when the compound is administered; however they are usually mild and evanescent. Recently, several patients taking carnitine have developed a drug-induced myasthenic syndrome. This condition disappeared four to five days after stopping the carnitine (De Grandis et al, 1980). Since it appears that steroids may enhance carnitine transport into muscle fibers (Milstad and Bihmer, 1979), and/or activate lipase (Avigan et al, 1983), prednisone (60 to 100 mg daily) should be given to patients who do not respond satisfactorily to carnitine therapy alone (Engel and Angelini, 1973). In addition, riboflavin may be of benefit in those who do not respond to carnitine and MCT oil (Carroll, 1981).

An illustrative case history follows.

Case Report

An 8-year-old boy was taken to his physician for evaluation of his "muscular dystrophy." The child, a product of a normal pregnancy, was slow to achieve his motor milestones and did not walk until age two. In school he was nicknamed "turtle" because he invariably lagged behind in all activities. The parents had discussed the problem with a neighbor whose son had muscular dystrophy. Told that there is no treatment for the disease, they were discouraged from seeking medical attention. Finally with the coaxing of the school nurse, the boy was brought to a physician.

Physical examination revealed intact mentation and cranial nerve function. Weakness and mild atrophy were present in the shoulder and hip girdles and proximal limb musculature. Gowers' sign was elicited. There was no muscle hypertrophy. Evaluation was initiated with measurement of serum muscle enzymes. The CPK was twice normal. Not convinced of the *parent's* diagnosis of muscular dystrophy, the physician arranged for a muscle biopsy. Because he was considering myositis, disorders of muscle energy metabolism, "congenital myopathies," as well as muscular dystrophy, special stains were requested (see Table 2-1). The muscle tissue appeared normal except that there were increased lipid droplets as seen with the oil red O stain. The patient was referred to a near-by neuromuscular disease center where he was found to have low levels of muscle carnitine (with normal serum levels). Treatment with carnitine and prednisone produced marked improvement. The neighbor's child is currently being evaluated by the same physician.

CARNITINE PALMITYL TRANSFERASE DEFICIENCY

In 1970, Engel et al described twin sisters who had intermittent episodes of painful muscle cramps frequently related to exercise and accompanied by the passage of dark brown urine. Biochemical studies failed to pinpoint the metabolic defect in these two patients. However the investigators correctly postulated a problem in the utilization of long chain fatty acids. Several years later, Di Mauro and Di Mauro (1973) described a similar patient who was shown to have a deficiency of the enzyme carnitine palmityl transferase (CPT). With the addition of subsequent case material, the clinical picture of this disorder became clarified. However, the diagnosis of CPT deficiency may be elusive because patients appear normal between attacks and frequently have normal muscle biopsies.

Clinical Presentation: Signs and Symptoms

Carnitine palmityl transferase deficiency is a disorder with an autosomal recessive pattern of inheritance. Typically, symptoms of muscle cramping and pain, followed by myoglobinuria appear in the first or second decade. Prolonged rather than strenuous activity characteristically precipitates an attack. Fasting prior to exercise increases the likelihood of an episode. Patients examined during an episode commonly demonstrate diffuse muscle swelling and tenderness. Strength is difficult to assess because of the extensive muscle discomfort but proximal limb weakness may be evident. Episodes generally last several hours to days. However, the muscle necrosis and myoglobinuria may be of a magnitude sufficient to precipitate acute renal failure. Between attacks patients are normal.

The patient with exercise-induced muscle pain and/or cramps should be evaluated for the possibility of a metabolic myopathy. Disorders of muscle glucose or lipid metabolism must be considered especially if the exercise provokes a rise in the serum CPK and myoglobinuria. While clinical features of the attacks may give clues as to the diagnosis (see Table 9-3), laboratory studies, including ischemic exercise test, fasting with determination of urine ketones, and muscle biopsy are needed.

Table 9-3. Comparison of CPT Deficiency and Myophosphorylase Deficiency

	CPT Deficiency	Myophosphorylase Deficiency
inheritance	aut. recessive	aut. recessive or dominant
exercise intolerance	with prolonged activity	with strenuous activity
exercise-induced myoglobinuria	yes	yes
fasting-induced myoglobinuria	yes	no
second wind phenomenon	no	yes
chronic myopathy as a later sequel	unknown	yes
ischemic exercise test	normal	abnormal
ketone production with fasting	abnormal	normal

Laboratory Studies

Blood studies

During an attack, serum muscle enzymes are usually elevated. In addition, patients with the disease commonly have persistently elevated serum triglycerides and cholesterol (Di Mauro and Eastwood, 1977).

Muscle biopsy

A normal muscle biopsy does not speak against the diagnosis of CPT deficiency. When possible, such biopsies should be performed around the time of an attack. Even when done under optimal conditions, however, the biopsy is frequently normal. The increase of lipid droplets especially in type I fibers, is the most commonly encountered abnormality. Muscle homogenates from patients with CPT deficiency show normal myophosphorylase, phosphofructokinase and carnitine levels. However, CPT activity is significantly reduced. Many patients demonstrate delayed or absent ketone body formation when subjected to a prolonged fast.

Other

Unlike myophosphorylase deficiency and other disorders of muscle carbohydrate metabolism, the ischemic exercise test is normal in CPT deficiency. Because the enzyme is also deficient in the liver, ketone production with prolonged fasting is usually delayed or absent.

Pathophysiology

During normal activity or brief periods of exercise, patients with CPT deficiency utilize serum glucose and muscle glycogen as energy substrates. After prolonged exercise, especially with some degree of fasting, muscle and liver glycogen stores are depleted. Because of the CPT deficiency, long chain fatty acids cannot enter mitochondria to be oxidized and thus the muscle's demands for ATP cannot be satisfied. As a result, there is weakness, muscle necrosis, and myoglobinuria.

Treatment

Treatment is aimed at providing the muscle with substrates that it can metabolize. Patients with the disorder should be instructed to ingest high carbohydrate foods or medium chain fatty acid supplements (Portagen) prior to anticipated prolonged activity (Cumming et al, 1976).

MYOADENYLATE DEAMINASE DEFICIENCY

In 1978, Fishbein et al reported myoadenylate deaminase (MADA) deficiency in a group of patients with no distinctive clinical features. They found this enzyme lacking in five of the 250 muscle biopsies surveyed. Because of the crucial role MADA plays in the purine nucleotide cycle (Tornheim and Lowenstein, 1974), it is not illogical to assume that its absence will cause significant neuromuscular dysfunction. However, since the initial reports of MADA deficiency, it has remained controversial as to whether the deficiency is a normal variant or a true disease state. Shumate et al (1979) screened 256 muscle biopsies from patients with a variety of neuromuscular complaints. They found MADA deficiency in six (2.3 percent). Of these six patients, two had exercise-induced myalgias and/or muscle fatigue. Several others were suffering from motor neuron disease. In the remaining two cases, one had a viral associated myositis while the other had evidence of an adult-onset dystrophy. The investigators concluded that MADA deficiency is common and is only a coincidental finding in patients with neuromuscular disease.

More recently Keleman et al (1982) reported several families with MADA deficiency, in whom exercise-induced myalgias, muscle swelling, and CPK elevations were the predominant clinical manifestations. Myoglobinuria was not part of the syndrome. All of the eight symptomatic family members had normal electrodiagnostic studies and muscle biopsies, but five of them lacked MADA activity by histochemical stains. Of the remaining three symptomatic family members, two had low levels of MADA as determined by biochemical analysis of their muscle tissue. None of the asymptomatic family members were found to be deficient in MADA. This same group of investigators reported that in their patients with neuromuscular symptoms other than myalgias, approximately one to two percent had MADA deficiency. However, in those with myalgias, over eight percent were lacking the enzyme. They concluded that MADA deficiency is responsible for a clinical syndrome characterized by exercise-induced muscle pain and fatigue and is not a laboratory abnormality in search of a disease. Further clarification of the MADA deficiency controversy is needed.

MITOCHONDRIAL MYOPATHIES AND "RAGGED-RED" FIBER DISEASE

The term mitochondrial myopathy is applied to a group of clinically heterogenous disorders that share in common structural and/or functional abnormalities of their mitochondria. The mitochondria in these diseases are unusually large, bizarre, and overly abundant. Many contain crystalline inclusions. With the light microscope some of the muscle fibers appear mottled red and have a course sarcoplasmic texture. These are alluded to as "ragged-red" fibers (see Figure 9-12).

Because this group of disorders is so diverse, classification is difficult. Perhaps the best organization of the mitochondrial myopathies appears in Walton's textbook of muscle disease.

One group of mitochondrial myopathies is characterized clinically by profuse diaphoresis, heat intolerance, asthenia, weakness, and elevated BMR. Loose coupling or uncoupling of oxidative phosphorylation appears to be the underlying problem. The mitochondria appear dysmorphic and contain abnormal inclusions. Cases have been described by Luft (1962), Afifi (1972), Schotland (1976) and their co-workers.

In a second group of patients there is a specific deficiency of one or more mitochondrial respiratory chain components. Included in this group are cases of cytochrome C oxidase deficiency, cytochrome B deficiency (Spiro et al, 1970), and NADH coenzyme Q reductase deficiency (Morgan-Hughes et al, 1979). Many of these patients exhibit clinical manifestations of diffuse neuronal dysfunction including dementia, ataxia, cranial and peripheral neuropathies as well as myopathy. A resting lactic acidemia and "ragged-red" fibers on biopsy are common. There is another group of patients with a similar clinical and laboratory picture but whose precise biochemical abnormality has not been ascertained. These patients are frequently referred to as cases of "ragged-red" fiber disease. They are discussed in further detail in the section that follows.

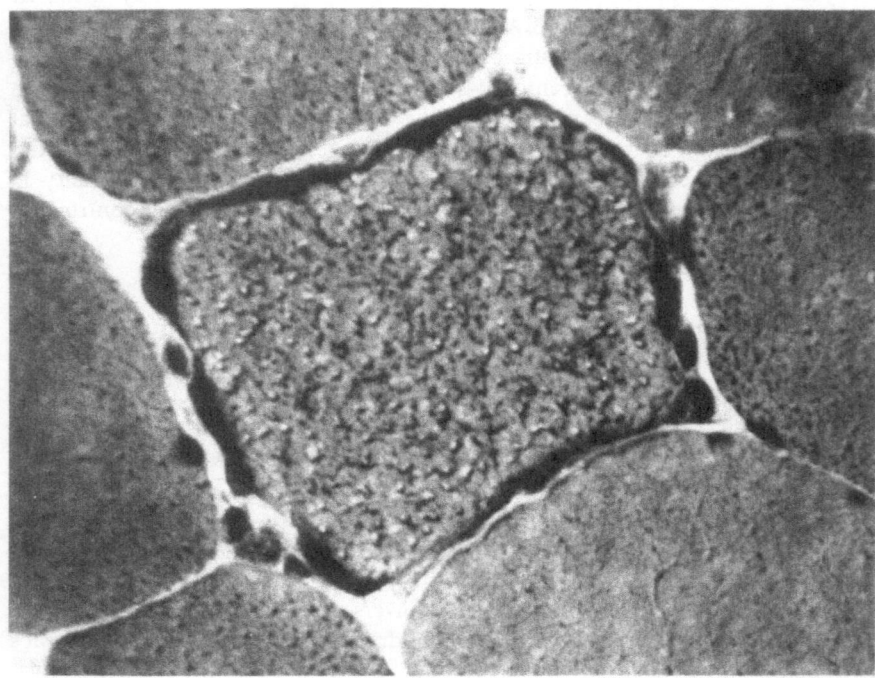

Figure 9-12. Muscle biopsy—ragged-red fiber disease (modified Gomori tri-chrome stain). A single "ragged-red" fiber is seen in the figure.

"RAGGED-RED" FIBER DISEASE (OCULOCRANIOSOMATIC NEUROMUSCULAR DISEASE, KEARNS-SAYRE SYNDROME)

The clinical combination of ophthalmoplegia beginning in childhood, atypical pigmentary degeneration of the retina, and heart block, was originally described by Kearns and Sayre in 1958. With additional case material it became apparent that this triad of symptoms may be seen in combination with other neurologic and endocrine abnormalities and the term "ophthalmoplegia plus" was applied to this group of disorders (Drachman, 1968). Common to almost all of these patients is a morphologic abnormality in a variable number of somatic muscle fibers. These aberrant fibers have a coarse, mottled appearance with the modified trichrome stain (Engel and Cunningham, 1963) and are called "ragged-red" fibers.

Clinical Presentation: Signs and Symptoms

With the exception of two patients (Schnitzler and Robertson, 1979), all cases of "ragged-red" fiber disease have been sporadic.

Typically, symptoms appear in early childhood or adolescence. Ptosis and/or ophthalmoplegia are the first of the diagnostic triad of signs to appear in over 90 percent of the cases (Berenberg et al, 1977). Reginal pigment degeneration and cardiac conduction abnormalities generally develop within ten years of onset of the extraocular muscle palsies. The pigmentary degeneration of the retina is characterized by a fine diffuse pattern of stippled pigment that is central in location, does not entail vascular changes, and rarely causes field cuts. Cardiac conduction defects include prolonged intraventricular conduction time, bundle branch block, and complete atrio-ventricular block. Eventually more than 90 percent of patients manifest ECG abnormalities. Such individuals are prone to Stokes-Adams attacks and sudden death.

Muscle fatigue with exercise is common and some patients have fixed mild proximal muscle weakness. Cranial musculature other than those governing ocular motility, may also be involved.

Other manifestations of the syndrome include short stature, delayed puberty, cerebellar signs, sensorineural hearing loss, mental retardation, and vestibular dysfunction.

Laboratory Studies

Patients with "ragged-red" fiber disease may be confused with cases of myasthenia gravis, oculopharyngeal dystrophy, myotonic atrophy, Refsum disease, and Bassen-Kornzweig syndrome. However, appropriate laboratory studies, electromyography, and muscle biopsy make the distinction less problematic.

Muscle biopsy

Oculocraniosomatic neuromuscular disease is characterized histologically by "ragged-red" fibers which make up between one and five percent of the total number. With the modified trichrome stain these fibers have excessive amounts of a course subsarcolemmal and intermyofibrillar red material (see Figure 9-12). Histochemical stains reveal that most "ragged-red" fibers are of the type I variety. In addition, they frequently demonstrate increased staining with oil red O, indicating excessive lipid accumulation within these fibers (Olson et al, 1972). Ultrastructurally, "ragged-red" fibers are found to contain increased numbers of mitochondria with morphologically abnormal cristae.

Electromyography

Approximately half of the patients with the disorder will have an EMG pattern characterized by *b*rief, *s*mall amplitude, *a*bundant, *p*olyphasic *p*otentials (BSAPPs). The absence of myotonia excludes myotonic atrophy from diagnostic consideration, and normal repetitive nerve stimulation studies weigh against myasthenia gravis. Absence of slowing of peripheral nerve conduction velocities makes Refum's disease and Bassen-Kornzweig unlikely diagnoses.

Cerebrospinal fluid and blood studies

One of the laboratory hallmarks of the disorder is an unexplained increase in the cerebrospinal fluid protein. This has been noted in virtually all cases and usually exceeds 70 mg percent.

In order to exclude Bassen-Kornzweig disease, serum lipoprotein electrophoresis as well as a blood smear (looking for acanthocytes) should be obtained.

Pathophysiology

"Ragged-red" fiber disease is a progressive degenerative disorder of unknown cause and pathogenesis. However, it has long been suspected that abnormal mitochondrial function is the basis of the disorder. In support of this theory is the observation that "ragged-red" fibers can be produced in animals given 2,4-dinitrophenol, a known uncoupler of mitochondrial oxidative phosphorylation (Melmed et al, 1975). In addition, several patients with the disease have had elevated serum levels of pyruvate and lactate, at rest and after exercise, suggesting a metabolic block in the oxidation of carbohydrates (Sulaiman et al, 1974).

Recently it has been found that such patients excrete abnormally large amounts of dicarboxylic acids. This implies disordered B-oxidation of long chain fatty acids within mitochondria (Blumenkopf et al, 1982).

Treatment

Presently there is no treatment for the disease. However, it is important to recognize these patients and to screen them for asymptomatic cardiac conduction problems. Early pacemaker insertion may be lifesaving. Furthermore, some patients with "ragged-red" fiber disease have a blunted ventilatory response to hypoxia and hypercapnea (Carroll et al, 1976). Such individuals should be warned about the potential hazards of high altitude travel and use of sedating drugs.

CHAPTER 10

Neuromuscular Manifestations
of Endocrine Dysfunction

ACROMEGALY

Acromegaly is a chronic disease of middle age characterized by the over-production of bone, connective tissue, and viscera in response to excessive secretion of adenohypophyseal growth hormone (GH). Early sumptoms are related to the peripheral effects of GH and, less commonly, to mechanical pressure of the intrasellar tumor mass. Paresthesias in the hands and feet secondary to mechanical entrapment of peripheral nerves and stiffness of the slowly expanding fingers and toes are early complaints. Later, there are obvious changes in the patient's physical appearance, along with headaches and visual impairment. Acromegalics may exhibit extraordinary muscle power and bulk during the early stages of their illness. With the passage of time, muscle weakness ensues, and finally there is muscle atrophy.

Clinical Presentation: Signs and Symptoms

Symptoms of muscle weakness with decreased exercise tolerance begin insidiously and usually appear 8 to 25 years after the onset of acromegaly. Pickett et al (1975) report that their patients with myopathy had symptoms of acromegaly for an average of eight years longer than those without muscle disease. Their observations suggest that the longer the patient is exposed to elevated GH levels, the more likely he is to develop myopathy. Furthermore, it seems that the length of time a patient is exposed to increased levels of GH is more significant than the actual levels of the hormone.

The myopathy is initially mild and produces a few symptoms. Patients may compalin of inability to complete routine activities without an increased number of rest periods, or may find that performing hard labor is impossible.

Proximal muscles including the deltoids, infraspinati, and iliopsoas muscles are the earliest and most severely affected. Cranial and axial muscles are characteristically spared. In the early stages, the muscles appear bulky and have a flabby texture. Later, atrophy of the proximal muscle groups is evident. At no time are there fasciculations, muscle tenderness, or changes in deep tendon reflexes. The myopathy is relentlessly progressive unless GH levels are reduced.

Laboratory Studies

Serum muscle enzymes

Muscle enzyme studies in patients with acromegaly are usually normal. Mastaglia et al (1970) found a modest elevation in the CPK levels in five out of eleven patients with acromegaly and muscle weakness, while Pickett et al (1975) observed a similar rise in only one of nine affected patients.

Electromyography and nerve conduction studies

Electromyographic abnormalities (i.e., BSAPP pattern) frequently precede clinical evidence of muscle disease in acromegaly. Nerve conduction studies may reveal multiple peripheral nerve entrapments with unilateral or bilateral carpal tunnel syndromes in approximately 50 percent of patients.

Muscle biopsy

Light miscroscopic findings in acromegalic myopathy include increased number of internal nuclei and increased glycogen particles. Histochemical stains reveal hypertrophy of type I and II fibers initially with selective type II atrophy at later stages (Mastaglia, 1973).

Degenerating mitochondria and increased numbers of lipofucsin bodies may be seen when such muscle is viewed under the electron microscope.

Pathogenesis

How growth hormone exerts its effect on the structure and function of muscle tissue is a question that has not as yet been answered. What is evident is that while GH does increase muscle bulk and protein content (at least initially), it does not enhance muscle performance. This has been demonstrated experimentally by Bigland and Jehring (1952) who administered GH to rats. They observed a 15 to 40 percent increase in muscle weight. However, these hypertrophied muscles actually produced fewer grams of tension per gram of muscle tissue than normal muscle.

Some studies have suggested that GH interferes with glycolytic pathways and muscle energy metabolism and that this plays a role in the mechanism of muscle weakness. They point to the increased amount of glycogen deposits in acromegalic muscle as supportive evidence.

Treatment and Prognosis

After treatment for acromegaly (either surgical removal of the tumor or radiation), the myopathy slowly and gradually improves. This improvement continues for approximately one to two years. After this time, whatever weakness remains probably represents a permanent deficit. There appears to be no correlation between the absolute serum levels of GH or the relative decline after treatment and the degree of recovery of muscle power.

HYPERPARATHYROIDISM

Bone disease, renal failure, kidney stones, peptic ulcers, and pancreatitis are among the more common manifestations of hyperparathyroidism. Although symptoms of fatigue and subjective weakness occur frequently, muscle atrophy with objective loss of motor power are less well-recognized features of the disease. Most studies indicate that between four and eight percent of patients with parathyroid hypersecretion have unequivocal loss of strength and wasting (Smith and Stern, 1967; Frame et al, 1968). Other studies have found true weakness in almost 90 percent of such patients (Patten et al, 1974). All agree that there is little correlation between the degree of neuromuscular involvement and the magnitude of change in the serum calcium and phosphorous concentrations.

Clinical Presentation: Signs and Symptoms

A form of neuromuscular disease characterized by wasting and weakness, especially in the proximal muscles of the limbs, has been observed in patients with primary hyperparathyroidism.

Migratory muscle pain and stiffness commonly precede by years the development of weakness and wasting. In most instances, loss of muscle power and bulk is evident initially in the proximal lower extremities and pelvic girdle. A waddling gait, difficulty climbing stairs, and arising from a squatting position are early disabilities noted by afflicted individuals. The weakness progresses at a variable rate, but in most cases ultimately involves the proximal upper limbs and shoulder girdle. Severity of the neuromuscular syndrome most closely correlates to the duration of the dysparathyroid state and not to the degree of Ca^{++}/PO_4 = abnormalities.

Because such patients often have hyperactive tendon reifexes, fine tremors of the tongue resembling fibrillations, and intact sensory function, they are sometimes mistaken for cases of amyotrophic lateral sclerosis. It is, therefore, imperative that all suspected cases of motor neuron disease be screened for parathyroid dysfunction.

Laboratory Studies

Serum muscle enzymes and blood studies

Serum CPK, aldolase and transaminases are normal in virtually all instances of hyperparathyroid neuromuscular disease. As would be expected, such individuals have elevated serum Ca^{++} levels, low serum PO_4 = concentration, calcuria, and increased PTH levels.

Electrodiagnostic studies

The most common electrical abnormality in patients with hyperparathyroidism and weakness is the BSAPP pattern. Such an EMG pattern is nonspecific and can be seen in both primary myopathic and neurogenic processes (see Chapter 2). The absence of evidence of active and chronic denervation (fibrillations, positive sharp waves, and large amplitude long duration motor units) helps to differentiate the condition from amyotrophic lateral sclerosis.

Muscle morphology

Histologic study of symptomatic muscle reveals normal tissue or mild neuropathic changes in most cases. None of the alterations which characterize a myopathic process (see Chapter 2) are evident.

Pathogenesis

The cause of the neuromuscular symptoms associated with hyperparathyroidism is unknown. However, it appears that the primary pathology involves the lower motor neuron rather than the muscle as was once believed. Since there is no correlation between the degree of Ca^{++}/PO_4 = abnormalities and the severity of the neuromuscular symptoms it is difficult to attribute the lower motor neuron dysfunction to deranged mineral metabolism.

Treatment and Prognosis

With treatment of the hyperparathyroid state (i.e., removal of the parathyroid adenoma) the majority of patients improve. Most of them report a feeling of increased energy and vitality and an enhanced muscle performance. Normal strength is regained in many cases, but the rate of improvement is variable and unpredictable.

HYPERTHYROIDISM

Thyroid hormones affect almost every aspect of bodily function and metabolism. Therefore it is not surprising that thyroid hypersecretion is known to produce a wide range of neurological dysfunction. Thyrotoxic myopathy, exophthalmic ophthalmoplegia, thyrotoxic periodic paralysis, myasthenia gravis and the Eaton-Lambert syndrome represent the currently recognized neuromuscular manifestations that occur in association with hyperthyroidism (Engel, 1972). In some instances, obvious systemic signs of thyrotoxicosis (i.e., palpitations, tremor, weight loss, and diarrhea) accompany the neuromuscular symptoms. At other times, the neurologic manifestations are the predominant presenting complaints, with other somatic evidence of thyroid dysfunction entirely absent.

In general, there is not a good correlation between the degree of chemical hyperthyroidism and the severity of the neuromuscular symptoms.

HYPERTHYROID MYOPATHY

Clinical Presentation: Signs and Symptoms

Approximately 60 percent of all patients with hyperthyroidism demonstrate clinical weakness and/or wasting. In five percent of these cases, muscle weakness is the presenting complaint and precedes by many months other symptoms of thyroid hypersecretion (Ramsay, 1968). Therefore one must always keep in mind the diagnosis of the "apathetic" hyperthyroidism as a possible cause of obscure muscle weakness.

While hyperthyroidism is predominantly a disease of females by a factor of seven, males account for over 25 percent of the cases of myopathy. Proximal muscle weakness alone occurs in three-quarters of affected patients, while a combination of proximal and distal involvement is seen in the remaining one-quarter. About 15 percent of cases will have evidence of bulbar muscle impairment including nasal speech and dysarthria. Spontaneous muscle "twitching" is noted in 20 percent of cases.

Some degree of muscle thinning is common in these patients and is in keeping with the generalized weight loss. Disproportionate proximal muscle wasting is apparent in less than ten percent of cases. The deep tendon relfexes are hyperactive or normal but rarely hypoactive. The myopathy of hyperthyroidism has a mean age of onset of 48 years and is usually seen in an elderly patient with unrecognized and/or untreated hyperthyroidism. The severity of the weakness and wasting correlates with the duration of the thyrotoxic state rather than with the degree of chemical dysthyroidism. The myopathy rarely has a fulminant onset within a few weeks of the development of overt thyrotoxicosis. Such cases are characterized by the sudden onset of bulbar palsy, generalized muscle weakness, prostration, and coma.

Laboratory Studies

Serum muscle enzymes and urine creatine

Serum creatine phosphokinase levels are normal or low in patients with hyperthyroid myopathy. Creatinuria is common but of uncertain significance.

Electromyography

Electromyographic studies of hyperthyroid patients are abnormal in over 90 percent of cases. Most frequently, a pattern of short duration (brief), low amplitude (small), abundant, polyphasic potentials (BSAPPs) are recorded from affected muscle. Occasionally, in the resting state, spontaneous trains of normal motor unit potentials occurring at a regular rate are seen. These are not fasciculations but are myokymic discharges. After correction of the hyperthyroid state, the EMG abnormalities usually disappear.

Muscle biopsy

Nonspecific morphologic alterations in the muscle are seen in a high percentage of cases of thyrotoxic myopathy. These alterations include fiber atrophy, edema, and a variable degree of cellular infiltration. Biochemical analysis of such muscle reveals low concentrations of ATP and creatine phosphate, the high energy compounds essential for muscle contraction (Satoyoshi et al, 1963).

Pathogenesis

There is good evidence that an excess of thyroid hormones produces a state of "loose" coupling of mitochondrial oxidative phosphorylation. This may be the underlying metabolic derangement responsible for hyperthyroid myopathy. Oxidative phosphorylation is that process by which the energy derived from redox reactions of the mitochondrial electron transport system is utilized for the formation of ATP (see Figure 9-4). One of the most important characteristics of oxidative phosphorylation is the phenomenon of respiratory control: that is, mitochondria oxidize substrates at less than maximal rates unless ADP and inorganic orthophosphate (Pi) are present. Therefore mitchondrial respiration is normally controlled by availability of ADP and Pi. If the process of oxidative phosphorylation is uncoupled, then oxidation (respiration) takes place in the absence of ADP and Pi. Furthermore, in the uncoupled state, even when ADP and Pi are present, the energy derived from the transfer of electrons is not utilized for the phosphorylation of ADP to ATP. As a result there is no net synthesis of ATP, and the energy produced is dissipated as heat. A state of "loose" coupling exists when oxidation of substrates procedes even in the absence of ADP and Pi, but the efficiency of ATP production when both are present may be abnormal. "Loose" coupling could explain the excess heat production and low levels of muscle ATP observed in the thyrotoxic state. However, other mechanisms may be responsible for hyperthyroid myopathy (Solemon et al, 1968).

Treatment and Prognosis

Complete recovery from the myopathy after control of the hyperthyroid state is the rule. Several weeks after the euthyroid state is reached, muscle power improves and over the ensuing months, reaches nearly normal levels.

EXOPHTHALMIC OPHTHALMOPLEGIA

An ocular myopathy, sometimes called exophthalmic ophthalmoplegia, occurs in four to fourteen percent of hyperthyroid patients (Krudrjaveev, 1978). Restricted eye movements secondary to dysthyroidism rarely occur before age 20 but dysthroidism is the most common cause of spontaneous diplopia in middle age and early senescence. The incidence of this ocular myopathy is unrelated to the occurrence or degree of skeletal myopathy.

The ophthalmoplegia is usually associated with exophthalmos, but it is unlikely that the latter is the cause of the impaired ocular motility (Schultz et al, 1960). In subtle cases, the striking clinical signs of congestive proptosis may be absent but spontaneous lid retraction or lid lag (von Graefe's sign) on downgaze is observable. Careful inspection of the globe may reveal dilated tortuous conjunctival vessels, and "jelly roll" edema of the lids. Limitation of elevation of the eyes is by far the most common disturbance. Although it mimics a superior rectus palsy, the actual problem is fibrotic shortening of the inferior rectus which restricts upward rotation. If both inferior recti are involved, the condition may resemble an upgaze paresis (midbrain syndrome). Medial rectus fibrosis with restricted abduction is the second most common abnormality followed by lateral rectus involvement. Limitation of elevation frequently occurs alone but it is rare for any other eye movement to be restricted in the presence of full elevation.

The ophthalmoplegia may appear during the hyperthyroid state but, more commonly, becomes manifest when the patient is euthyroid. The diagnosis is not difficult on clinical grounds if the physician searches for concomitant ocular signs and uses the forced duction test (see Figure 10-1). In addition, a computerized tomographic scan of the orbits may be of help in confirming the

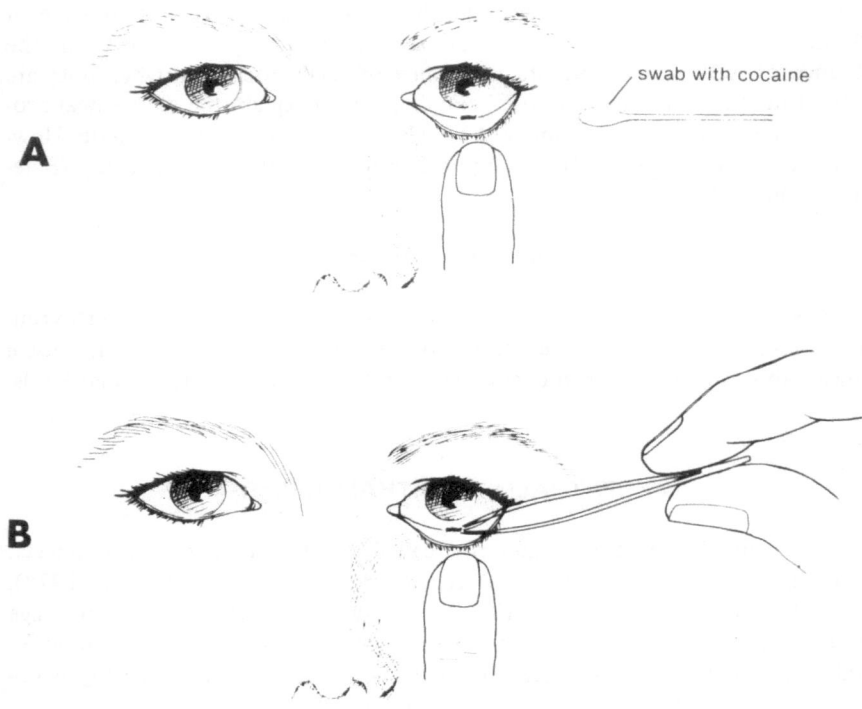

Figure 10-1. The forced duction test. Using 10% cocaine, the insertion of the muscle in question (i.e., inferior rectus) is anesthetized (A). The muscle insertion in then grasped with forceps and an attempt is made to manually rotate the globe upwards (B).

presence of abnormally thickened fibrotic extra ocular muscles. If the forced duction test is negative and the movements of the globe are not mechanically restricted, an edrophonium test (see Figure 3-8), repetitive nerve stimulation studies, and acetycholine receptor antibody titers are needed in order to exclude myasthenia gravis. Muscle biopsy is also indicated to rule out "ragged-red" fiber disease. Because a carotid cavernous fistula may produce symptoms and signs indistinguishable from Graves' ophthalmopathy, careful auscultation over the orbits is essential. A bruit discovered in this setting is supportive of a fistulous communication.

Chemical assessment of thyroid function is often of little diagnostic value. Ocular manifestations may antedate or postdate laboratory evidence of thyroid hypersecretion. According to one study, approximately 28 percent of patients first recognize the existence of eye disease within 18 months before, and another 28 percent after, the date when hyperthyroidism was diagnosed. In 24 percent, the eye manifestings and hyperthyroidism are recognized simultaneously, In the remaining group of patients, hyperthyroidism is *never* documented (Gorman 1983). At the time of ocular symptoms most patients are chemically euthyroid.

Histologic examination of involved muscles in exophthalmic ophthalmoplegia show them to be edematous and infiltrated with lymphocytes. In addition, mucopolysaccharide deposits beneath the sarcolemmal membrane of muscle fibers have also been described.

Dysthyroid ophthalmoplegia is a self-limiting disease. The ocular paresis reaches its maximum in a few months, then subsides or stabilizes. Less than 50 percent achieve complete recovery. Correction of the abnormal thyroid state does not seem to alter the natural course of the disorder. Steroid therapy is of no benefit. The use of prisms and surgical correction of the strabismus may be of benefit (Scott and Thalacker, 1981).

THYROTOXIC PERIODIC PARALYSIS (TPP)

Hyperthyroidism may be associated with episodic recurrent attacks of weakness clinically identical to those of primary hypokalemic periodic paralysis (see Chapter 7). The incidence of TPP in hyperthyroidism is about two percent (Kudrjaveev, 1978). Most of the patients are males of oriental or Mexican origin. Attacks of periodic paralysis may antedate other manifestations of thyrotoxicosis by months or years (Ali, 1975).

TPP resembles primary hypokalemic periodic paralysis in many respects. In both, generalized attacks tend to affect proximal muscles before distal ones, and to spare the cranial nerves and diaphragm. The serum potassium level falls during these episodes. Meals high in carbohydrate content or sodium, cold exposure, or exercise followed by rest, provoke attacks. Urinary retention and oliguria may accompany the episodes. Unlike primary hypokalemic periodic paralysis, TPP is much more common in males, is not familial, and is cured when the hyperthyroid state is corrected. In addition, the development of a permanent fixed vacuolar myopathy after many attacks of the primary hypokalemic variety does not occur in TPP.

MYASTHENIA GRAVIS AND THE EATON-LAMBERT
SYNDROME IN THYROTOXICOSIS

Less than one percent of hyperthyroid patients develop the clinical and electrical characteristics of myasthenia gravis (see Chapter 3). On the other hand, the occurrence of thyrotoxicosis in myasthenia gravis is estimated to be about five percent (Osserman et al, 1967). Almost 80 percent of patients in whom the two diseases coexist are female. Correction of the hyperthyroid state is followed by improvement of the myasthenia in the majority of cases.

The association between hyperthyroidism and myasthenia is a curious one and may be explained by an altered immune state in these patients. However, a direct effect of thyroid hormones on neuromuscular junction transmission can also explain their common occurrence (Hoffman and Denys, 1972). The Eaton-Lambert syndrome may also be associated with hyperthyroidism (Mori and Takamori, 1976).

HYPOTHYROIDISM

Hypothyroidism (myxedema) is about one-eighth as common as hyperthyroidism; over 80 percent of cases are female. Symptoms and signs develop insidiously over many years and are often vague and non-specific. Because the early complaints of fatigue, sluggishness, apathy, and dry skin are frequently passed off as part of a depressive illness, many cases go untreated for years. Neurologic manifestations are common in hypothyroidism and include acroparesthesias, polyneuropathy, mononeuropathies (especially carpal tunnel syndrome), dementia and ataxia. A variety of neuromuscular syndromes may also accompany myxedema including myopathy, a syndrome resembling myasthenia gravis, and the Eaton-Lambert syndrome. In addition, patients with myxedema may complain of muscle cramps and exhibit myoedema. These phenomena may occur singly or in any combination and may be of varying severity.

Myoedema, sometimes referred to as the "mounding phenomenon" is the immediate local ridge of contracted muscle that appears when the muscle is tapped briskly with a reflex hammer. Typically, the mound lasts for 30 to 60 seconds and is electrically silent (Salick and Pearson, 1967). Myoedema is seen in 30 to 60 percent of hypothyroid patients. However, it is not specific for myxedema but may also occur in various states of malnutrition (i.e., sprue and carcinoma).

Pseudomyotonic reflexes occur in a high percent of patients with hypothyroidism. Such reflexes are slow to contract and relax, and differ from true myotonia in which only the relaxation phase is slow. In addition, true myotonia is characterized electrically by high frequency repetitive discharges which show a recurrent variation of the frequency and amplitude. Pseudomyotonic discharges show no such variation.

Clinical Presentation: Signs and Symptoms

Subjective complaints of weakness are universal among patients suffering from myxedema. However, objective evidence of diminished strength is apparent in approximately 25 percent of such individuals and takes several forms.

Almost 20 percent of hypothyroid children exhibit weakness and generalized muscle hypertrophy (Kocher-Debré-Sémélaigne syndrome) (Najjar, 1974). Such children have a Herculean appearance with the most striking hypertrophy involving the lower extremities, particularly the gastrocnemius muscles. Typically the syndrome occurs in boys with long-standing untreated hypothyroidism. A similar illness rarely appears in adults (Hoffman syndrome) but these adult patients, unlike their pediatric counterparts, usually have prominent pseudomyotonia and muscle cramps. In both child and adult cases, girdle muscles are weaker than distal ones. Ocular and bulbar musculature typically are not involved.

Because of the prominent increase in muscle mass and the accompanying muscle pain, these patients may be mistaken for cases of myotonia congenita. With the aid of laboratory studies (i.e., thyroid functions, serum CPK levels, and electrical studies) the differentiation should not be troublesome.

More commonly, adults with hypothyroid myopathy do not exhibit increased muscle girth but instead manifest weakness, stiffness, cramps, and myoedema. In some of these patients, muscle stiffness and pain constitute the major complaints. Such cases clinically mimic polymyositis or one of the myotonias. Cold weather worsens the stiffness and pain. Phenylbutazone aggravates these symptoms rather than relieves them as it does in other rheumatic conditions (Golding, 1970). Variable degrees of hip and should girdle weakness are seen in these individuals. Ptosis is a prominent component in some.

Laboratory Studies

Serum muscle enzymes

Striking elevations in the serum CPK are characteristic of hypothyroid myopathy. Such increases range from two to six times normal (Hochberg et al, 1976) and may cause the unwary physician to misdiagnose the conditions as polymyositis. Thyroid function tests should be performed on all patients presenting with symmetric proximal muscle weakness and elevated muscle enzymes. With treatment of the hypothyroid state CPK level return to normal.

Electrodiagnostic studies

Electromyographic abnormalities are found in over 70 percent of patients with hypothyroidism (Rao et al, 1980). Needle electromyography of proximal muscles most frequently reveals a BSAPP pattern (see Chapter 2). Fibrillation potentials and sharp waves are not usually seen, which is a help in differentiating these cases from imflammatory muscle disease. As previously discussed, percussion myoedema is electrically silent while pseudomyotonia is characterized by spontaneous bizarre discharges without the waxing and waning qualities of true myotonia.

Muscle biopsy

There are no consistent histologic changes in the muscles of patients with hypothyroid myopathy. In many instances, the muscle is morphologically normal while in other cases, there may be nonspecific abnormalities, including abnormal glycogen inclusions, type II fiber atrophy, increased numbers of internal nuclei, vacuoles, and necrotic fibers (McKeran et al, 1980).

Pathogenesis

No hypothyroid patient has as yet been reported as having autoanitbodies to muscle. In view of this and the fact that most patients have complete recovery on thyroid replacement, it is unlikely that autoimmunity is an etiologic factor in the myopathy. Most likely the myopathy results from inadequate amounts of thyroid hormone and the subsequent disordered energy production at the subcellular level (i.e., mitochondria).

Treatment

With restoration of euthyroidism, the majority of patients improve and many return to their premorbid state. As the patient improves, serum CPK levels decrease.

MYASTHENIA GRAVIS AND EATON-LAMBERT
SYNDROME WITH HYPOTHYROIDISM

The occurrence of myasthenia gravis with hypothyroidism is less frequent as compared to its association with hyperthyroidism. Evaluation of thyroid function in several large groups of myasthenic patients reveal that two to five percent will have chemical evidence of inadequate thyroid hormones (Osserman et al, 1967). Clinically, the myasthenia associated with hypothyroidism may not respond to anticholinesterase drugs. However, almost all cases improve with appropriate treatment of the hypothyroid state.

The facilitating neuromuscular syndrome (Eaton-Lambert syndrome) has also been described in association with hypothyroidism.

CHAPTER 11

Toxic Myopathies

ALCOHOL MYOPATHY

Until recently, it was not widely appreciated that muscle disease occurs in association with alcoholism. However, as early as the middle of the nineteenth century, clinicians realized that neurogenic disease alone could not explain all the motor symptoms manifested by their alcoholic patients.

It is now recognized that a spectrum of muscle disease exists in alcoholics. Perkoff (1971) in his review, concluded that there are at least three distinct clinical forms of alcohol myopathy, each with a unique course and symptom complex. These are outlined below:

1. subclinical myopathy
2. acute alcohol myopathy
   a. abrupt onset
   b. subacute onset
3. chronic alcohol myopathy

It should be emphasized that while these are distinct clinical entities, they actually represent progressive stages in a common pathologic process (see Figure 11-1).

Clinical Presentation: Signs and Symptoms

Subclinical alcohol myopathy

Evidence of a subclinical form of alcohol myopathy rests on the demonstration of increased serum levels of enzymes derived from muscle tissue and other laboratory abnormalities. These patients are asymptomatic with regard to motor complaints, and biochemical abnormalities indicative of muscle damage are discovered only serendipitously.

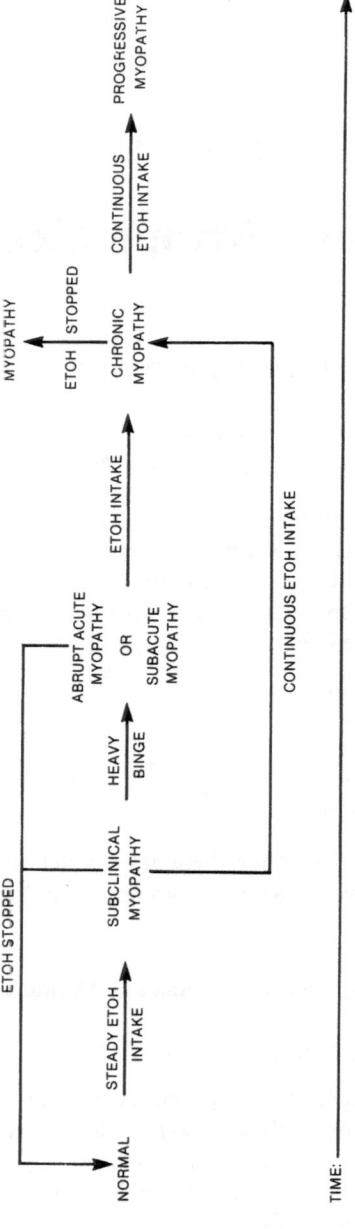

Figure 11-1. Natural history of muscle disease in alcoholism.

Acute alcohol myopathy

This variety of alcoholic muscle disease can be subdivided into two diverse subgroups. The first type usually follows close upon a recent episode of binge drinking. Characteristically, there is an abrupt onset of severe muscle pain and swelling, myoglobinuria, and fever. The muscle discomfort and tenderness are most pronounced in the lower extremeities, especially the calves and quadriceps groups. Even the lightest touch may produce exquisite pain and therefore manual muscle testing for evaluation of strength is often impossible. Palpable muscle edema is also a hallmark of the acute alcoholic muscle syndrome. When localized to the calves, as is commonly the case, it can lead even the most astute clinician to the erroneous diagnosis of acute thrombophlebitis. The findings of other stigmata of excessive alcohol intake (i.e., jaundice, hepatomegaly, tremulousness, nystagmus, ataxia, peripheral neuropathy) together with the characteristic laboratory abnormalities make the correct diagnosis more evident. It is important that these patients be carefully observed for signs of acute renal failure. The accompanying rhabdomyolysis with myoglobinuria is frequently of sufficient magnitude to produce this potentially fatal sequela.

A less common subtype of acute alcohol myopathy has been described by Perkoff et al (1967) and others. This syndrome usually evolves over a two to three week period and produces progressive diffuse muscle weakness. Muscle edema with tenderness and gross myoglobinuria do not occur.

Chronic alcohol myopathy

Chronic myopathy is a common sequela of severe prolonged alcohol abuse. It is usually seen in patients over 30 years of age. Some of these patients have had previous episodes of acute alcohol myopathy whereas other progress slowly from the subclinical to the chronic form. The major complaints in this group reflect proximal muscle weakness. Climbing stairs, squatting, and raising the arms above the horizontal plane become increasingly more difficult. Examination reveals diffuse muscle weakness and atrophy. However, the most severely affected muscles are those of the shoulder and hip girdles, upper arms and thighs. Characteristically, the facial and oropharyngeal muscles are spared, but the striated muscle of the upper esophagus may be rarely involved, with a subsequent dysphagia (Weber et al, 1981).

Alcoholic cardiomyopathy may be present at this stage, but more frequently, skeletal myopathy and cardiomyopathy occur separately. Patients with the chronic myopathy picture invariably show systemic signs of long-standing overindulgence.

Laboratory Studies

Serum muscle enzymes

Serum levels of muscle enzymes aid the clinician in diagnosing alcohol myopathy. Different stages of the myopathy have characteristic patterns of enzyme abnormalities.

Despite the absence of motor manifestations, 60 percent of patients following a severe alcohol debauch will have elevated serum levels of creatine phosphokinase (CPK). These levels steadily decrease once the patient stops drinking and become normal by the fifth to seventh day of abstinence.

It is in the acute form of alcohol myopathy with rhabdomyolysis that the enzyme elevations are most pronounced. Creatine phosphokinase levels of 100 times normal are not uncommon. Other sarcoplasmic enzymes (GOT, GPT, LDH, and aldolase) are elevated two to ten times their expected values. Gross myoglobinuria is evident by the brown discoloration of the patient's urine.

In the chronic form serum muscle enzyme determinations reflect low grade muscle damage. All of the above mentioned enzymes are mildly elevated approximately two to four times above normal. Persistent creatinuria accompanies this form of alcohol myopathy.

Electromyography

Electromyography may demonstrate "myopathic" changes (i.e., BSAPP pattern), However, it is more common to encounter abnormalities compatible with both muscle and peripheral nerve disease (axonal neuropathy) in these patients.

Ischemic exercise test

The ischemic exercise test, as previously described (see Figure 9-9), is abnormal in all stages of the alcohol myopathy syndrome. Afflicted patients show impaired lactic acid production with ischemic exercise, similar to patients with myophosphorylase deficiency (McArlde's disease). Recently, Chui et al (1978) demonstrated that this abnormality could be reproduced in normal subjects who were given a single oral load of ethanol, suggesting that this impaired production may not be a feature of alcohol myopathy but rather merely a reflection of ethanol intake.

Muscle biopsy

It is under the microscope that the continuous spectrum of the alcohol myopathy syndrome becomes most apparent. Serial biopsies demonstrate the relentless progression of muscle damage in the chronic imbiber. The acute stages of alcohol myopathy are characterized histopathologically by fiber necrosis, fiber swelling, and sarcoplasmic vacuolation. As the disease process continues, damaged fibers are replaced by fibrous tissue and fat. Regenerating fibers also become numerous. A more complete description of the histologic changes in the myopathy is available (Klinkerfuss et al, 1967).

Pathogenesis

The pathogenesis of the alcohol myopathy syndrome is unknown. Poor nutrition per se is not the primary cause as was once believed but it probably does play a contributary yet minor role. Currently, the most widely accepted theories postulate that ethanol is directly toxic to muscle tissue. Alcohol may disrupt the sarcolemmal membrane and/or inhibit the Na,K-ATPase pump. This could explain the pathologic findings of increased sarcoplasmic water and deranged electrolyte concentrations in muscle fibers of alcoholics. Alcohol has also been shown to impair both calcium release from the sarcoplasmic reticulum and the binding of calcium by troponin (Rubin 1979). Such alterations may greatly impede the contractile process.

Impaired glycolysis resulting from depression of myophosphorylase activity has also been proposed. Altered levels of Krebs cycle intermediates and the abnormal ischemic exercise tests in chronic imbibers are supportive of this theory. Finally, hypokalemia (Rubenstein and Wainapel, 1977) and hypophosphatemia have also been implicated in the pathogenesis of the disorder.

Course

Common to all stages of the alcohol myopathic syndrome is the fact that improvement will occur if ethanol abuse is abandoned. In the acute stages, recovery is rapid if total abstinence is adhered to. In two to three weeks most patients recover fully. The remainder will improve substantially to a point, then stabilize with residual proximal muscle weakness. In the chronic stages of the disease, cessation of drinking will similarly result in improvement. However, this improvement is much slower and is never complete. These patients improve for up to six months after complete abstinence. After six months, whatever motor deficit remains probably represents a permanent disability.

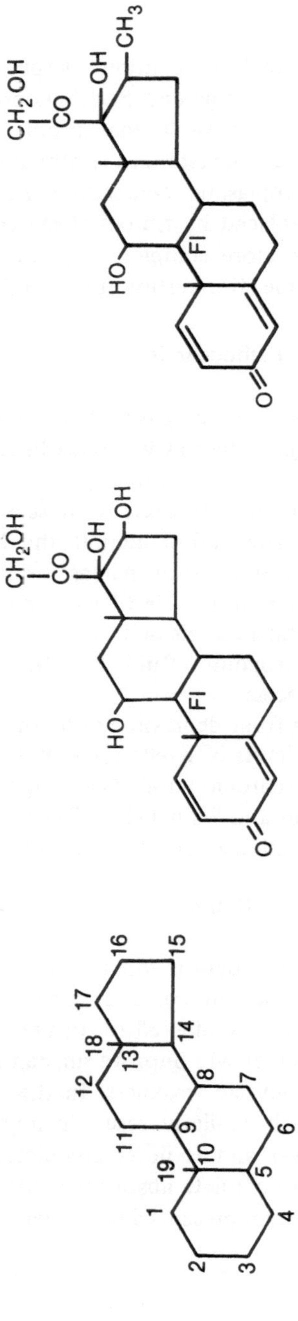

Figure 11-2. Chemical structure of steroids.

STEROID ATROPHY

Steroid compounds are widely prescribed in clinical medicine today, mainly because of their anti-inflammatory properties. Although the therapeutic value of these compounds in undeniable, approximately one-third of all patients taking corticosteroids will develop serious complications necessitating the cessation of therapy.

Muscular weakness and wasting have been reported as untoward side effects of steroid treatment but these have been overshadowed by the other more common features of hyperadrenocorticism. The first reported case of steroid-induced weakness occurred in a patient receiving triamcinolone (Dubois, 1958). It soon became evident that this toxic manifestation was not limited to triamcinolone but could occur with the use of a wide variety of related compounds. Dexamethasone, prednisone, prednisolone, cortisone and ACTH have all been implicated as potential myopathic agents. Overall, approximately seven percent of patients receiving steroids will develop some degree of muscle weakness (Askari et al, 1976); however, the rate of incidence varies with the type of steroid preparation used. The preparations with an alpha fluoro configuration such as triamcinolone and dexamethasone (see Figure 11-2) have the greatest tendency to produce muscle disease (Faludi et al, 1966). Taken together, these two compounds account for over two-thirds of the reported cases of steroid atrophy.

Surprisingly, susceptibility to corticosteroid-induced weakness does not seem to be related to the age of the patient, the underlying connective tissue disease, the magnitude of dose, or the duration of maintenance therapy. The majority of patients developing steroid-induced muscle weakness receive between 5,000 and 15,000 mg. of prednisone or its equivalent (see Table 11-1). The time of onset of weakness relative to the introduction of steroids is also variable, occurring most often within five months of the initiation of treatment.

Table 11-1. Steroid Equivalents

	Anti-Inflammatory Potency	Na^+ Retaining Potency	Equivalents (mg)
cortisol	1.0	+2	25
hydrocortisone	0.8	+2	20
prednisone	3.5	+1	5
prednisolone	4.0	+1	5
triamcinolone	5.0	0	4
dexamethasone	30.0	0	0.75

Clinical Presentation: Signs and Symptoms

Weakness attributed to steroids occurs in all age groups. The greatest incidence seems to be between the third and fifth decades but this probably reflects the prevalence of steroid treated conditions in this group.

The onset of weakness is typically insidious but in about one-fourth of patients it occurs suddenly, evolving over a period of a few days. Muscle weakness and atrophy is generally symmetric with initial involvement of the proximal muscle groups of the lower extremities. Difficulty in climbing stairs and rising from a squatting position are the most common early complaints. The shoulder girdles and distal extremities become progressively involved. Muscles supplied by cranial nerves, sphincteric muscles, and cardiac muscles are generally spared. Myalgias are common and are often a prominent component of the disorder. Deep tendon reflexes are preserved and sensory abnormalities are not encountered. If the condition goes unrecognized, the patient may become totally incapacitated and bedridden.

The patient in whom steroid atrophy develops frequently demonstrates other undesirable side effects of the drug. These include Cushingoid facies, osteoporosis, psychiatric disorders (euphoria or depression), diabetes and/or hypertension. The common association of osteroporosis and steroid atrophy is particularly noteworthy. These two conditions occur together at such a high frequency that it has been stated that any patient receiving steroids who develops severe osteoporosis should be suspected of harboring a hidden steroid myopathy.

Laboratory Studies

Serum muscle enzyme

Serial determinations of serum muscle enzymes are extremely helpful in deciding whether an increase in muscle weakness occurring during steroid treatment of connective tissue disease is because of an exacerbation of the disease or is a result of the therapy. These enzymes are usually elevated with a flare-up of polymyositis, but are invariably normal with steroid-induced weakness. An increase in strength as the steroids are withdrawn is further supportive evidence of a drug related myopathy.

Electromyography

Electromyographic studies in steroid atrophy may be normal but more commonly reveal "myopathic" (BSAPP pattern) or neuromyopathic changes. Coomes (1965) found that by doing serial EMG studies on his rheumatoid patients who were taking steroids he could predict which ones would develop myopathy. A reduction in the duration of the motor unit potential appeared to be a warning of incipient myopathy.

Muscle biopsy

Histologic study of muscle tissue is helpful in differentiating steroid-induced weakness from inflammatory muscle disease. Under the light microscope the former is characterized by fiber atrophy. The atrophy is selective for type II fibers (Askari et al, 1976) (see Figure 11-3). Large vacuolated mitochondria are frequently seen with the electron microscope. These changes are non-specific and may occur with prolonged bed rest and pyramidal tract disease. However, the absence of inflammatory infiltrates speaks against an active myositic process.

Pathogenesis

The pathogenesis of steroid atrophy is not yet understood. The catabolic effect of steroids on proteins is well known and this might be the mechanism of the myopathy. Cortisol, the prototype glucocorticoid hormone promotes hepatic gluconeogenesis from amino acids derived from extra-hepatic protein. Thus, severe protein wasting resulting in osteoporosis and myopathy will occur at high non-physiologic glucocorticoid levels. Synthetic steroids, especially those with a fluorine group, have heightened anti-inflammatory actions. These analogues do not dissociate the anti-inflammatory effects from the catabolic action on proteins, and these compounds, therefore, have the greatest tendency to induce weakness.

Other studies (Vignos et al, 1973) have postulated that steroid-induced muscle weakness is related to inhibition of myophosphorylase activity and/or oxidative respiration in muscle tissue.

Treatment and Prognosis

Steroid atrophy is a reversible condition if adequately treated. Proper treatment consists of either gradual withdrawal of steroids, reduction in dosage without discontinuing the drug, or substitution of one steroid compound for another. Triamcinolone has been substituted with prednisone or prednisolone in equivalent doses with complete reversal of the weakness. (Dubois, 1958; Williams, 1959). (Surprisingly, the substituted steroids themselves have been implicated in other cases of myopathy.) Improvement can begin as early as three days and as late as five weeks after the institution of treatment. Myalgias disappear prior to improvement in muscle strength. Complete recovery within two to twelve months is the general rule.

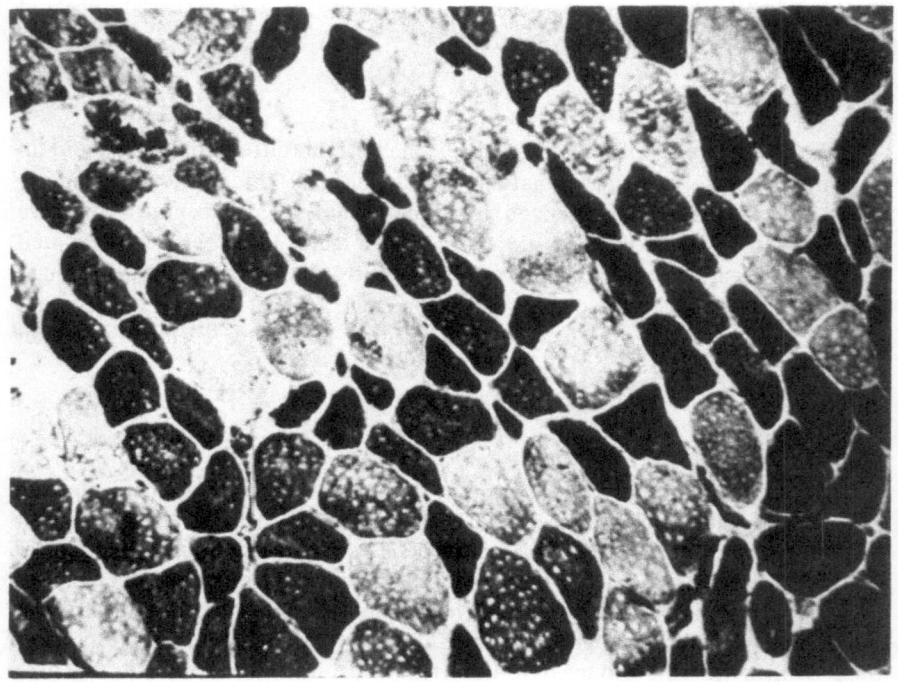

Figure 11-3. Muscle biopsy—steroid atrophy (ATP-ase Stain, pH 94). Note the numerous small dark (type II) fibers. The "vacuoles" are freeze artifact.

Case Report

A 43-year-old woman complained of diffuse weakness, muscle and joint pains for six months. Examination revealed weakness in a proximal distribution with preserved cranial nerve function and deep tendon reflexes. Blood tests including thyroid functions, serum Ca^{++}/PO_4, and CPK were ordered and she was found to have a CPK level eight times normal. A biopsy was organized and was compatible with inflammatory muscle disease. Treatment was initiated with 50 mg of daily prednisone for three weeks. This was changed to 100 mg every other day over the next 20 days (see Case 2, Chapter 3). After six weeks of therapy, her strength improved and CPK levels fell to three times normal. She did well over the next four months and it was decided to taper her steroid dose by 5 mg decrements every three or four weeks. Four months later (prednisone dose 70 mg Q.O.D.) she noted increased fatigue and weakness in her lower extremities. In addition, persistent back pain had developed. She was re-evaluated by her physician who found extreme proximal muscle weakness and atrophy, and X-ray evidence of osteopenia. Suspecting an exacerbation of her myositis, the physician increased the prednisone to 100 mg Q.O.D. However, the patient deteriorated further and was hospitalized. In the hospital, serial CPK's were found to be 1.5 to 2 times normal putting the diagnosis of active myositis in doubt. A repeat muscle biopsy was arranged which showed little evidence of active inflammatory disease but prominent type II fiber atrophy consistent with steroid myopathy. The prednisone dose was rapidly reduced to 50 mg Q.O.D. and physical therapy initiated. Her strength gradually returned over the next two weeks and she was discharged. The plan is to taper her prednisone by 5 mg decrements every three or four weeks and follow her disease activity will be monitored with monthly examinations and CPK determinations.

CHLOROQUINE MYOPATHY

Chloroquine first came into use during World War II as an antimalarial suppressive and prophylactic. Since that time, it has been administered in the treatment of other diseases including amoebic hepatitis, discoid and systemic lupus erythematosus, rheumatoid arthritis, periarteritis nodosa, and sarcoidosis. While the ocular toxicity of the drug was recognized early by its pioneer users, it wasn't until 1963 (Whisnant et al) that its myopathic effects were first appreciated. These early reports attributed the drug-induced weakness to both nerve and muscle damage. More recent studies on experimental animals verify the deleterious effects of the drug on muscle tissue.

Aguayo et al (1970) administered chloroquine phosphate to rabbits and successfully induced severe weakness in these animals. Complete autopsy studies were performed in all cases and pathologic changes were observed only in skeletal and cardiac muscle. The central and peripheral nervous systems were strikingly free of abnormalities. In human subjects, this is not as easily demonstrated because many of the diseases in which chloroquine is used have neuropathy as part of the disease state.

Clinical Presentation: Signs and Symptoms

Evidence of chloroquine toxicity, either ocular or muscular, usually does not appear until the patient has been taking the drug at least six months. The total amount ingested before symptoms appear varies widely from 45 to 1,100 g. Because excretion of the drug is slow and continues for months or years after its administration has ceased, the effect of a prolonged course of the drug is cumulative. Therefore, even low doses, when taken over long periods of time, are potentially toxic.

The general clinical picture is that of a progressive proximal myopathy with the lower extremities affected earlier and more severely than the upper limbs. While Hughes et al (1971) report a case of chloroquine myopathy involving the bulbar muscles and producing dysphagia, this is not a frequent occurrence. Cardiac involvement is extremely common and often severe enough to produce congestive heart failure. In about half the cases with myopathy there will be signs and symptoms of ocular toxicity. These include reversible corneal opacities and irreversible pigmentary macular changes with loss of central visual acuity. Sensory complaints, muscle tenderness and cramps are absent.

Laboratory Studies

Serum muscle enzymes

While the disease is active, serum muscle enzyme levels may be abnormal. With cessation of the drug, these levels will return to normal in four to six months.

Electromyography

Patients taking chloroquine may exhibit EMG abnormalities compatible with both neuropathic and "myopathic" disease.

Muscle biopsy

The most conspicuous light miscroscopic finding in chloroquine myopathy is fiber degeneration characterized by abundant granular deposits and vaculations (see Figure 11-4). Special histochemical staining techniques reveal that type I fibers are selectively and more severely affected than type II cells. The granular deposits are PAS positive and are located both centrally and peripherally in the diseased fibers. This PAS positive material, suggestive of glycogen deposits, is also found within the vacuoles. Necrotic fibers are rarely seen. Electron microscopic studies show prominent changes in sarcoplasmic mitochondria. These organelles appear disrupted, and several may be enclosed within an electron dense membrane. Such mitochondrial aggregates are sometimes referred to as "myelin figures" because of their superificial resemblance to degenerating meylin sheaths. Cardiac muscle exhibits similar changes.

Pathogenesis

As yet, the pathogenesis of chloroquine myopathy has not been fully unraveled. Smith and O'Grady (1966) proposed that chlorquine's therapeutic

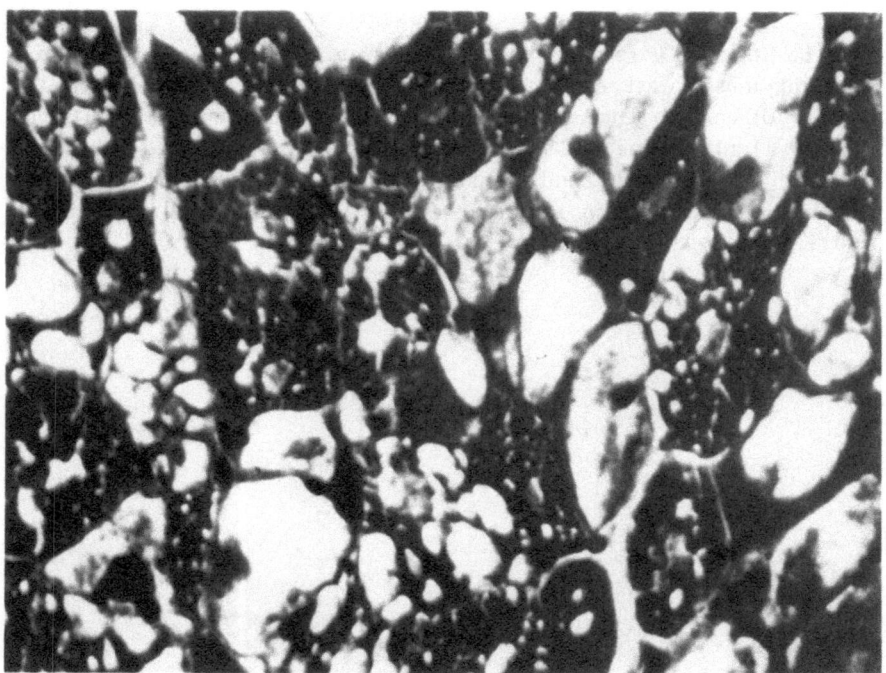

Figure 11-4. Muscle biopsy—chloroquine myopathy. Extensive vacuolar changes characterize the biopsy.

value in malaria is related to its high affinity for hemoglobin in red blood cells. Type I fibers have higher concentrations of myoglobin than type II fibers and it is felt that this could explain the drug's preferential toxicity to the oxidative fiber type. Other have postulated that the drug interferes with enzymes in glycogen utilization and point to the characteristic granular glycogen deposits in affected muscle tissue as supportive evidence.

Course and Treatment

In most toxic myopathies, improvement will occur if the offending agent is withdrawn. Chloroquine myopathy is no different and most patients show evidence of improvement approximately two to three months after the drug is stopped. Accompanying the clinical improvement is a return of the serum muscle enzymes to normal levels.

OTHER TOXIC MYOPATHIES

The literature is speckled with isolated case reports of a variety of drugs producing muscle weakness. Included in this list of drugs are vincristine (Bradley et al, 1970), emetine (Duane and Engel, 1970), colchicine (Markand and D'Agostino, 1971), nitroxoline (O'Grady and Smith, 1966), polymyxin E (Van Haeverbeek, Ectors, Van Haelst, and Franken, 1974), clofibrate (Smith, MacFie and Oliver, 1970), penicillamine (Schraeder et al, 1972), and epsilon amino-caproic acid (Kennard et al, 1980).

References

Afifi, A., Ibraheim, M., Bergman, R., et al. 1972. Morphologic features of hypermetabolic mitochondrial disease. J. Neurol. Sci. 15: 271.

Afifi, A., Smith, J., Zellweger, H. 1965. Congenital nonprogressive myopathy. Central core disease and nemaline myopathy in one family. Neurology 15: 371–381.

Aguayo, A., Hudgson, P. 1970. Observations on the short-term effects of chloroquine on skeletal muscle. J. Neurol Sci. 11: 301–325.

Aita, J. 1973. Neurologic worm diseases. Nebr. Med. J. 58: 408–410.

Aldrich, M., Yong, K., Sanders, D. 1979. Effects of D-penicillamine on neuromuscular transmission in rats. Muscle and Nerve 2: 180–185.

Ali, K. 1975. Hypokalemic periodic paralysis complicating thyrotoxicosis. Brit. Med. J. 4: 503-504.

Angelini, C., Engel, A. G. 1972. Comparative study of acid maltase deficiency. Arch. Neurol. 26: 344–349.

Angelini, C., Lucke, S., Cantarutti, F. 1976. Carnitine deficiency of skeletal muscles: report of a treated case. Neurology 26: 633–637.

Argov, Z., Mastaglia, F. 1979. Disorders of neuromuscular transmission caused by drugs. NEJM 301: 409–413.

Arundell, F., Wilkinson, R., Haserick, J. 1960. Dermatomyositis and malignant neoplasms in adults. Arch. Dermatol. 82: 772–775.

Askanas, V., Engel, W. K., Reddy, N., 35 al. 1979. X-linked recessive congenital muscle fiber hypotrophy with central nuclei. Arch. Neurol. 36:604–609.

Askari, A., Vignos, P., Moskowitz, R. 1976. Steroid myopathy in connective tissue disease. Am. J. Med. 61: 485–492.

Avigan, J., Askansas, V., Engel, W. K. 1983. Muscle carnitine deficiency: Fatty acid metabolism in cultured fibroblasts and muscle cells. Neurology 33: 1021–1026.

Barchi, R. 1975. Myotonia. Arch. Neurol. 32: 175–180.

Barnes, B. 1976. Dermatomyositis and malignancy. Ann. Intern. Med. 84:68-76.

Barr, R. 1966. Human trichinosis. Can. Med. Ass. J. 95: 912–917.

Barth, P., Wijngaarden, G., Bethlen, J. 1975. X-linked myotubular myopathy with fatal neonatal asphyxia. Neurol. 25: 531–536.

Barwick, D., Walton, J. 1963. Polymyositis. Am. J. Med. 35: 646, 660.

Baxter, D., Dyck, P. 1961. Paramyotonia congenita. Canad. Med. Assoc. J. 85: 113–118.

Beck, J., Davies, J. 1976. *Medical Parasitology*, St. Louis: C. V. Mosby.

Berenberg, R. Pellock, J., DiMauro, S., et al. 1977. Lumping or splitting; Oph-
thalmoplegia-plus or Kearns-Sayre syndrome. Ann. Neurol. 1: 37–54.
Bertagnolio, B., DiDonato, S., Peluchetti, D., et al. 1978. Acid maltase defici-
ency in adults. Eur. Neurol. 17: 193–205.
Bever, C., Aquino, A., Penn. A., et al. 1983. Prognosis of ocular myasthenia,
Ann. Neurol. 14: 516–519.
Bigland, B., Jehring, B. 1952. Muscle performance in rats, normal and treated
with growth hormone. J. Physiol. 116: 129–136.
Bishop, A., Gallup, B., Skeate, Y., et al. 171. Morphological studies on normal
and diseased human muscle in culture. J. Neurol. Sci. 13: 333–350.
Blumenkopf, B., Fales, H., Engel, W. K., Galdi, A. P. April 1982. Correlation
of fat tolerance test, decarboxylic aciduria and serum carnitine levels in a
family with carnitine deficiency. Presented at the Academy of Neurology,
34th annual meeting, Washington, D.C.
Bohan, A., Peter, J. 1975. Polymyositis and dermatomyositis. NEJM 929:
344–346, 403–407.
Bonilla, E., Schotland, D. 1970. Histochemical diagnosis of muscle phospho-
fructokinase deficiency. Arch. Neurol. 22: 8–12.
Bosch, E., Gowans, J., Munsat, T. 1979. Inflammatory myopathy in oculopharyngeal dystrophy. Muscle & Nerve 2: 73–77.
Botero, D., Castaño, S. 1982. Treatment of cysticercosis with praziquantel in
Columbia. Am. J. Trop. Med. Hyg. 31: 810–821.
Bradley, W. 1969. Adynamia episodica hereditaria. Brain 92: 345–378.
Bradley, W., Jones, M., Mussini, J-M. et al, 1978. Becker-type muscular dys-
trophy. Muscle & Nerve 1: 111–132.
Bradley, W., Lassman, L., Pearce, G., Walton, J. 1970. The neuromyopathy of
vincristine in man. Clinical electrophysiological and pathological studies.
J. Neurol. Sci. 10: 107–131.
Brain, R., Henson, R. 1958. Neurological syndromes associated with carcinoma.
Lancet 2: 971–975.
Bresolin, N., Ro, Y., Reyes, M. et al. 1983. Muscle phosphoglycerate mutase
(PGAM) deficiency: A second case. Neurology 33: 1049–53.
Brillman, J., Pincus, J. 1973. Myotonia periodic paralysis improved by negative
sodium balance. Arch. Neurol. 29: 67–69.
Brooke, M. 1973. *Muscle Biopsy: A Modern Approach*. London-Philadelphia-
Toronto. W. B. Saunders Co.
Brooks, J. 1969. Hyperkalemic periodic paralysis. Arch. Neurol. 20: 13–18.
Brown, H., Chattpadhyag, S., Patel, A. 1967. Erythrocyte abnormality in human
myopathy. Sci. 157: 1577-1578.
Brown, J., Nelson, J., Herrmann, C. 1968. Sjogren's syndrome with myopathic
and myasthenic features. Bull. La. Neurol. Soc. 33: 9.
Brownell, A., Gilbert, J., Shaw, D., et al. 1978. Adult-onset nemaline myopathy.
Neurology 28: 1306–1310.
Brungger, U., Kaeser, H. 1977. Paramyotonia congenita without cold paralysis
and myotonia levior. Eur. Neurol. 15: 2–4.
Burke, D., Skuse, N., Lethlean, K. 1974. An analysis of myotonia in paramyo-
tonia congenita. JNNP 37: 900–906.
Carlson, R. 1975. The possible role of cyclic AMP in neurotrophic control of
skeletal muscle. J. Physiol. 247: 343–361.
Carroll, J., Brooke, M., DeVivo, D., et al. 1978. Biochemical and physiologic

consequences of carnitine palmityl transferase deficiency. Muscle & Nerve 1: 103–108.

Carroll, J., Shumate, J., Brooke, M., Hagberg, J. 1981. Riboflavin-responsive lipid myopathy and carnitine deficiency. Neurology 31: 1557–1559.

Carroll, J., Zwillich, C., Wei, J., et al. 1976. Depressed ventilatory response in oculocraniosomatic neuromuscular disease. Neurology 26: 140–146.

Castleman, B. 1966. The pathology of the thymus gland in myasthenia gravis. Ann. N.Y. Acad. Sci. 135: 496–503.

Chad, D., Goud, P., Adelman, L., et al. 1982. Inclusion-body myositis associated with Sjögren's syndrome. Arch. Neurol. 39: 186–188.

Cherington, M. 1974. Botulism. Arch. Neurol. 30: 432–437.

Cherington, M., Ryan, D. 1970. Treatment of botulism with guanidine. NEJM 282: 195–197.

Cherington, M., Snyder, R. 1968. Tick paralysis. NEJM 278: 95–97.

Chou, S-M. 1967. Myxovirus-like structures in a case of human chronic polymyositis. Science 158: 1453–1455.

Christianson, H., Brunsting, L., Perry, H. 1956. Dermatomyositis: Unusual features, complications and treatment. Arch. Dermatol. 74: 581–589.

Chui, L., Munsat, T. 1976. Dominant inheritance in McArdle's syndrome. Arch. Neurol. 33: 636–641.

Chui, L., Munsat, T., Craig, J. 1978. Effect of ethanol on lactic acid production by exercised normal muscle. Muscle & Nerve 1: 57–61.

Clements, M., Hamilton, D., Siklos, P. 1981. Thyrotoxicosis presenting with choreoathetosis and severe myopathy. J. R. Soc. Med. 74: 459-460.

Cornelio, F., DiDonato, S., Peluchetti, D., et al. 1977. Fatal case of lipid storage myopathy with carnitine deficiency. JNNP 40: 170–178.

Crews, J., Kaiser, K., Brooke, M. 1976. Muscle pathology of myotonia congenita. J. Neurol. Sci. 28: 449–457.

Cumming, W., Hardy, M., Hudgson, P., et al. 1976. Carnitine palmityl transferase deficiency. J. Neurol. Sci. 30: 247–258.

Dalakas, M., Engel, W. K. 1983. Treatment of permanent muscle weakness in familiar hypokalemic periodic paralysis. Muscle & Nerve 6: 182–186.

Danieli, G., Angelini, C. 1976. Duchenne carrier detection. Lancet 2: 415–416.

Danon, M., Reyes, M., Perurena, O. 1982. Inclusion body myositis, Arch. Neurol. 39: 760–764.

Dau, P. 1980. Plasmapheresis therapy in myasthenia gravis. Muscle & Nerve 3: 468–482.

Dau, P. 1981. Plasmapheresis in idiopathic inflammatory myopathy. Arch. Neurol. 38: 544–552.

Dau, P., Denys, E. 1982. Plasmapheresis and immunosupressive drug therapy in Eaton-Lambert syndrome. Ann. Neurol. 11: 570–575.

Davis, M., Cilo, M., Plaitakis, A., Yahr, M. 1976. Trichinosis: severe myopathic involvement with recovery. Neurology 26: 37–40.

Delaney, P. 1977. Neurologic manifestations of sarcoidosis. Ann. Intern Med. 87: 336–345.

Demos, J. 1961. Mesure des temps de circulation chez 79 myopathies. Rev. Fr. Etud. Clin. Biol. 6: 876–887.

Denborough, M., Dennett, X., Anderson, R. 1973. Central core disease and malignant hyperthermia. Brit. Med. J. 1: 272-273.

Desmedt, J., Borenstein, S. 1977. Double-step stimulation test for myasthenic block: sensitization of postactivation exhaustion by ischemia. Ann. Neurol. 1: 55–64.

De Grandis, D., Mezzina, C., Fiaschi, A., et al. 1980. Myasthenia due to carnitine treatment. J. Neurol. Sci. 46: 365–371.

DeVere, R., Bradley, W. 1975. Polymyositis: Its presentation, morbidity and mortality. Brain 98: 637–666.

Di Donato, S., Peluchetti, D., Rimoldi, M., et al. 1980. Ketogenic response to fasting in human carnitine deficiencies. Clinica Chimica Acta 100: 209–214.

Di Mauro, S., Dalakas, M., Mirand, A. 1983. Phosphoglycerate kinase deficiency: another cause of recurrent myoglobinuria. Ann. Neurol. 13: 11–19.

Di Mauro, S., Di Mauro, P. 1973. Muscle carnitine palmityl transferase deficiency and myoglobinuria. Science 182: 929–931.

Di Mauro, S., Eastwood, A. 1977. Disorders of muscle glycogen and lipid metabolism. Adv. Neurol. 17: 123–142.

Di Mauro, S., Hartlage, P. 1978. Fatal infantile form of muscle phosphorylase deficiency. Neurology 28: 1124–1129.

Di Mauro, S., Miranda, A., Olarte, M. 1982. Muscle phosphoglycerate mutase deficiency. Neurology 32: 584–591.

Di Mauro, S., Stern, L., Mehler, M., et al. 1978. Adult-onset acid maltase deficiency: a postmortem study. Muscle & Nerve 1: 27–36.

Di Mauro, S., Trevisan, C., Hays, A. 1980. Disorders of lipid metabolism in muscle. Muscle & Nerve 3: 369–388.

Dluhy, R., Lauler, D., Thorn, G. 1973. Steroid therapy. Med. Clin. North Am. 57: 1155–1165.

Donadio, J., Gangarosa, E., Faich, G. 1971. Diagnosis and treatment of botulism. J. Infect. Dis. 124: 108–112.

Drachman, D. 1968. Ophthalmoplegia-plus. Arch. Neurol. 18: 654–674.

Drachman, D. 1978. Myasthenia Gravis. NEJM 298: 136–142.

Drachman, D., Adams, R., Josefek, L., Self, S. 1982. Functional activities of autoantibodies to acetycholine receptors and the clinical severity of myasthenia gravis. NEJM 307: 769–775.

Drachman, D., Angus, C., Adams, R. et al. 1978. Myasthenic antibodies crosslink acetylcholine receptors to accelerate degradation. NEJM 298: 1116–1122.

Duane, D., Engel, A. 1970. Emetine myopathy. Neurology 20: 733.

Dubois, E. 1958. Triamcinolone in the treatment of systemic lupus erythematosus. JAMA 167: 1590–1599.

Dubowitz, V., Brooke, M. 1973. *Muscle Biopsy: A Modern Approach.* Philadelphia: W. B. Saunders.

Dyck, P., Oviatt, K., Lambert, E. 1981. Intensified evaluation of referred unclassified neuropathies yields improved diagnosis. Ann. Neurol. 10: 222–226.

Dyken, M., Zeman, W., Rusche, T., 1969. Hypokalemic periodic paralysis. Neurology 19: 691–699.

Dyken, P. 1962. Sarcoidosis of skeletal muscle. Neurology 12: 643–651.

Edwards, R. H., et al. 1979. Muscle breakdown and repair in polymyositis. Muscle & Nerve 2: 223–228.

Eison, A., Berry, K., Gibson, Gillian. 1983. Inclusion body myositis (IBM): Myopathy or neuropathy. Neurology 33: 1109–1114.

Ellis, F., Keaney, N., Harriman, D., et al. 1972. Screening for malignant hyperthermia. Brit. Med. J. 1: 272-273.

Elmqvist, D., Lambert, E. 1968. Detailed analysis of neuromuscular transmission in a patient with myasthenic syndrome sometimes associated with bronchogenic carcinoma. Mayo Clin. Proc. 43: 689-713.

Emery, A., Clark, E., Simon, S., et al. 1967. Detection of carriers of benign X-linked muscular dystrophy. Br. Med. J. 4: 522-523.

Emmons, P., McLennan, H. 1959. Failure of acetylcholine release in tick paralysis. Nature 183: 474-475.

Eng, G., Epstein, B., Engel, W. K., et al. 1978. Malignant hyperthermia with central core disease with congenital dislocating hips. Arch. Neurol. 35: 189-197.

Engel, A. 1972. Neuromuscular manifestations of Graves' disease. Mayo Clin. Proc. 47: 919-925.

Engel, A., Angelini, C. 1973. Carnitine deficiency of human skeletal muscle with associated lipid storage myopathy. A new syndrome. Science 179: 899-902.

Engel, A., Banker, B., Eiben, R. 1977. Carnitine deficiency: clinical, morphological and biochemical observations in a fatal case. JNNP 40: 313-322.

Engel, A. G., Lambert, E. 1969. Calcium activation of electrically inexcitable muscle fibers in hypokalemic periodic paralysis. Neurology 19: 851-858.

Engel, A. G., Lambert, H., Gomez, M. 1977. A new myasthenic syndrome with end-plate acetylcholinesterase deficiency, small nerve terminals, and reduced acetylcholine release. Ann. Neurol. 4: 315-330.

Engel, A., Lambert, E., Mudder, D., Torres, C., Sahashi, K., Bertorini, T., Whitaker, J. 1982. A newly recognized congenital myasthenic syndrome attributed to a prolonged open time of the acetylcholine-induced ion channel. Ann. Neurol. 11: 553-569.

Engel, A. G., Santa, T. 1971. Histometric analysis of the ultrastructure of the neuromuscular junction in myasthenia gravis and in the myasthenic syndrome. Ann. N.Y. Acad. Sci. 183: 46-63.

Engel, A., Siekert, K. 1972. Lipid storage myopathy responsive to prednisone. Arch. Neurol. 27: 174-181.

Engel, W. K. 1975. Brief, small, abundant motor-unit action potentials. Neurology 25: 173-176.

Engel, W. K. 1976. Myasthenia gravis, corticosteroids and anticholinesterases. Ann. N.Y. Acad. Sci. 274: 623-630.

Engel, W. K. 1977. In Goldensohn, E., Appel, S. (eds). *Scientific approaches to clinical neurology*. Philadelphia: Lea and Febiger, pp. 1572-1600.

Engel, W. K., Brooke, M., Nelson, P. 1966. Histochemical studies of denervated or tenotomized cat muscle. Ann. N.Y. Acad. Sci. 138: 160-185.

Engel, W. K., Cunningham, G. 1963. Rapid examination of muscle tissue. An improved trichrome method for fresh-frozen biopsy sections. Neurology 13: 919-923.

Engel, W. K., Cunningham, G. 1970. Alkaline phosphatase–Positive abnormal muscle fibers of humans. J. Histochem. Cytochem. 18: 55-57.

Engel, W. K., Eyerman, E., Williams, H. 1963. Late-Onset type of skeletal muscle phosphorylase deficiency. NEJM 268: 135-137.

Engel, W. K., Gold, G., Karpati, G. 1968. Type I fiber hypotrophy and central core nuclei. Arch. Neurol. 18: 435-444.

Engel, W. K., Karpati, G. 1968. Impaired skeletal muscle maturation following neonatal neurectomy. Dev. Biology 17: 713–723.

Engel, W. K., Lichter, A., Galdi, A. P. 1981. Polymyositis: remarkable response to total body irradiation. Lancet 1: 658.

Engel, W. K., REsnick, J. 1966. Late-onset rod myopathy: A newly recognized acquired and progressive disease. Neurology 16: 308-309.

Engel, W. K., Vick, N., Glueck, C., et al. 1970. A skeletal muscle syndrome associated with intermittent symptoms and a possible defect of lipid metabolism. NEJM 282: 697–704.

Falk, G., Landa, J. 1960. Effects of potassium on frog skeletal muscle in chloride deficient medium. Am. J. Physiol. 198: 1225.

Faludi, G., Gotlieb, J., Meyers, J. 1966. Factors influencing the development of steroid myopathy. Ann. N.Y. Acad. Sci. 138: 61–78.

Fambrough, D., Drachman, D., Satyamurti, S. 1973. Neuromuscular junction in myasthenia gravis: decreased acetylcholine receptors. Science 182: 293–295.

Feigenbaum, J., Munsat, T. 1970. The neuromuscular syndrome of scapuloperoneal distribution. Bull. La. Neurol. Soc. 35: 47–57.

Feit, H., Brooke, M. 1976. Myophosphorylase deficiency: Two different molecular etiologies. Neurology 26: 963–967.

Fishbein, W., Armbrustmacher, V., Griffin, J. 1978. Myoadonylate deaminase deficiency: a new disease of muscle. Science 200: 545-548.

Fon, G., et al. 1982. Computed tomography of the anterior mediastinum in myasthenia gravis. Radiology 142: 135–141.

Frame, B., Heinze, E., Block, M., et al. 1968. Myopathy in primary hyperparathyroidism. Ann. Intern. Med. 68: 1022–1027.

Frank, J., Harati, Y., Butler, I., et al. 1980. Central core disease and malignant hyperthermia syndrome. Ann. Neurol. 7: 11–17.

Gabow, P., Keaney, W., Kelleher, S. 1982. The spectrum of rhabdomyolysis. Medicine 61-141-152.

Galdi, A. P. 1978. Essentials in the management of myasthenia gravis. Am. Fam. Phys. 17: 95–102.

Gallant, E., Aher, C., 1983. Malignant hyperthermia: Response of skeletal muscles to general anesthesia, Mayo Clin. Proc. 58: 758-763.

Gamstrop, I. 1956. Adynamia episodica hereditaria. Acta Paediat. 45: 108.

Gamstorp, I., et al. 1956. Adynamia episodica hereditaria. Am. J. Med. 23: 385–390.

Gardner-Thorpe, C. 1972. Muscle weakness due to sarcoid myopathy. Neurology 22: 917–928.

Gilhus, N., Aarli, J., Matre, R. 1984. Myasthenia gravis: Difference between thymoma-associated antibodies and cross-striational skeletal muscle antibodies, Neurology 34: 246-249.

Glaser, J. S. 1978. *Neuro-ophthalmology*. New York: Harper and Row.

Goldbert, S., Stern, L., Feldman, L., et al. 1982. Serial two-dimensional echocardiography in Duchenne muscular dystrophy. Neurology 10: 1101–1105.

Golding, D. 1970. Hypothyroidism presenting with musculoskeletal symptoms. Ann. Rheum. Dis. 29: 10–14.

Goodgold, J., Eberstein, A. 1978. Electrodiagnosis of Neuromuscular Diseases. Baltimore: Williams and Wilkins

Gomez, J., Engel, A., Dewald, G. 1977. Failure of inactivation of Duchenne dystrophy X-chromosome in one of female identical twins. Neurology 27: 537-541.

Gordon, A., Green, J., Lagonoff, D. 1970. Studies on a patient with familial hypokalemic periodic paralysis. Am. J. Med. 48: 185-195.

Gorman, C. 1982. Temporal relationship between onset of Graves' ophthalmopathy and diagnosis of throtoxicosis. Mayo Clin. Proc. 58: 515-519.

Gray, D., Morse, B., Phillips, W. 1962. Trichinosis for neurologic and cardiac involvement. Ann. Intern. Med. 57: 230-244.

Griggs, R. 1977. The myotonic disorders and the periodic paralysis. Adv. Neurol. 17: 143-159.

Griggs, R., Engel, W. K., Resnik, J. 1970. Acetazolamide treatment of hypokalemic periodic paralysis. Ann. Intern. Med. 73: 39-48.

Griggs, R., et al. 1978. Effects of acetazolamide on myotonia. Ann. Neurol. 3: 531-537.

Grob, D., Bonner, N., Namba, T. 1981. The natural course of myasthenia gravis and effect of therapeutic measures. Ann. N.Y. Acad. Sci. 377: 652-669.

Gronert, G. 1980. Malignant hyperthermia. Anesthesiology 53: 395-423.

Gutmann, L. 1972. The Eaton-Lambert syndrome and autoimmune disorders. Am. J. Med. 53: 354-356.

Gutmann, L., Pratt, L. 1976. Pathophysiologic aspects of human botulism. Arch Neurol. 33: 175-179.

Hagenan, R., Muller-Jensen, A. 1978. Botulism: Clinical neurophysiological findings. J. Neurol. 217: 159-171.

Hall, E. 1983. Direct effects of glucocorticoids on neuromuscular function, Clin. Neuropharm. 6: 169-183.

Hansotia, P., Frens, D. 1981. Hypersomnia associated with alveolar hypoventilation in myotonic dystrophy. Neurology 31: 1336-1337.

Harper, P. 1975. Congenital myotonic dystrophy in Britain. Arch. Dis. Child 50: 505-521.

Harper, P., Dyken, P. 1972. Early-onset dystrophia myotonica. Lancet 2: 53.

Harper, P., Johnston, D. 1972. Recessively inherited myotonia congenita. J. Med. Genet. 9: 213-215.

Hart, Z., Chang, C., Di Mauro, S., et al. 1978. Muscle carnitine deficiency and fatal cardiomyopathy. Neurology 28: 147-151.

Hartzell, H., Kuffler, S., Yoshikami, D. 1976. The number of acetylcholine molecules in a quantum and the interaction between quanta at the sub-synaptic membrane of the skeletal neuromuscular synapse. Cold Spring Harbor Symp. Quant. Biol. 40: 175-186.

Hathaway, P., Engel, W. K., Zellweger, H. 1970. Experimental myopathy after arterial embolization. Comparison with childhood X-linked pseudohypertrophic muscular dystrophy. Arch. Neurol. 22: 365-377.

Hochberg, M., Koppes, G., Edwards, C., et al. 1976. Hypothyroidism presenting as a polymyositis-like syndrome. Arth. Rheum. 19: 1363-1366.

Hoffman, S., Guthrie, T. 1975. Cerebral cysticercosis. South. Med. J. 68: 105-108.

Hoffman, W., Denys, E. 1972. Effect of thyroid hormones at the neuromuscular junction. Am. J. Physiol. 223: 283-287.

Hopkins, L., Jackson, J., Elsas, L. 1981. Emery-Dreifuss humoperoneal muscular dystrophy: An X-linked myopathy with unusual contractures and brady-cardia. Ann. Neurol. 10: 230–237.

Hosking, G., Cavanagh, N., Smyth, D., et al. 1977. Oral treatment of carnitine myopathy. Lancet 1: 853.

Hughes, J., Esiri, M., Oxbury, J., Whilty, C. 1971. Chloroquine myopathy. Q. J. Med. 40: 85–93.

Hughes, R., Park, D., Parsons, M., et al. 1971. Serum creatine kinase studies in detection of carriers of Duchenne dystrophy. JNNP 34: 527–530.

Huxley, H. 1969. The mechanism of muscle contraction. Science 164: 1356–1366.

Huxley, H., Hanson, J. 1954. Changes in the cross striations of muscle during contraction and stretch and their structural interpretation. Nature 173: 973–976.

Isaacs, H. 1961. A syndrome of continuous muscle fiber activity. JNNP 24: 319–325.

Ishikawa, K., et al. 1977. A neuromuscular transmission block produced by a cancer tissue extract derived from a patient with the myasthenic syndrome. Neurology 27: 140–143.

Jacob, J., Mathew, N. 1968. Pseudohypertrophic myopathy in cysticercosis. Neurology 18: 767–771.

Jacquemin, P., Van Hoof, F., Hers, H. 1973. Enzyme replacement in Pompe's disease. Birth Defects 9: 184–190.

Jenzer, G., et al. 1975. Autonomic dysfunction in botulism B: A clinical report. Neurology 25: 150–153, 1975.

Jolly, S., Pallis, C. 1971. Muscular pseudohypertrophy due to cysticercosis. J. Neurol. Sci. 12: 155–162.

Kanno, T., Sudo, K., Takeuchi, I. et al, 1980. Hereditary deficiency of lactate dehydrogenase M-subunit. Clin. Chim. Acta. 108: 267–276.

Kao, I., Gordon, A. 1977. Alteration of skeletal muscle cellular structures by potassium depletion. Neurology 27: 855–860.

Karpati, G., Carpenter, S., Engel, A., et al. 1975. The syndrome of systemic carnitine deficiency. Neurology 25: 16–24.

Katz, B., Miledi, R. 1973. The binding of acetylcholine to receptors and its removal from the synaptic cleft. J. Physiol. 231: 549–574.

Kazakov, V., Bogoredinsky, D., Znoyko, Z., et al. 1974. The facio-scapulolimb (or the facioscapulohumeral) type of muscular dystrophy. Eur. Neurol. 11: 236–260.

Kearns, T., Sayre, G. 1958. Retinitis pigmentosa, esternal ophthalmoplegia and complete heart block. Arch. Ophthmol. 60: 280–289.

Keleman, J., Rice, D., Bradley, W. G. et al. 1982. Familial myoadenylate deaminase deficiency and exertional myalgia. Neurology 32: 857–863.

Kelly, J., Daube, J., Lennon, V., Howard, F., Younge, B. 1982. The laboratory diagnosis of mild myasthenia gravis. Ann. Neurol. 12: 238–242.

Kennard, C., Swash, M., Henson, R. 1980. Myopathy due to epsilon amino caproic acid. Muscle & Nerve 3: 202–206.

Kim, C., Yamada, S. 1974. Myotonia congenita. Hawaii Med. J. 33: 15–18.

Klinkerfuss, G., Bleisch, V., Dioso, M., Perkoff, G. 1967. A spectrum of myopathy associated with alcoholism (Part II). Ann. Intern. Med. 67: 493–510.

Kramer, M., Aita, J. 1972. Trichinosis with central nervous system involvement. Neurology 22: 485–491.

Kudrjaveev T. 1978. *Neurologic Complications of Thyroid Dysfunction.* Adv. Neurol. Vol. 19., New York: Raven Press, pp. 619–636.

Kuhn, E., Fein, W., Schroder, J., et al. 1979. Early myocardial disease and cramping myalgia in Becker-type muscular dystrophy. A kindred. Neurology 29: 1144–1149.

Kumamoto, T., Fukuhara, N., Nagashima, M., et al. 1983. Distal myopathy. Arch. Neurol. 39: 367–371.

Layzer, R. 1982. Periodic paralysis and the sodium potassium pump. Ann. Neurol. 11: 547–552.

Layzer, R., Rasmussen, J. 1974. The molecular basis of muscle phosphofructo-kinase deficiency. Arch. Neurol. 31: 411–417.

Layzer, R., Rowland, L., Ranney, H. 1967. Muscle phosphofructinase deficiency. Arch. Neurol. 17: 512–523.

Lehman-Horn, F., Rudel, R., Dengler, R. et al, 1981. Membrane defects in paramyotonia congenita with and without myotonia in a warm environment. Muscle & Nerve 4: 396–406.

Lewis, R., Sumner, A. 1982. The electrodiagnostic distinctions between chronic familial and acquired demyelinative neuropathies. Neurology 32: 592–596.

Leyburn, P., Walton, J. 1960. Effects of changes in serum potassium upon myotonia. JNNP 23: 119–126.

Liveson, J., Spielholz, N. 1979. Peripheral Neurology: Case Studies in Electrodiagnosis. Philadelphia: F. A. Davis

Long, C., Haller, R., Foster, D., McGarry, J. 1982. Kinetics of carnitine-dependent fatty acid oxidation: implications for human carnitine deficiency. Neurology 32: 663–666.

Luft, R., Ikkos, D., Palmieri, G. et al. 1962. A case of severe hypermetabolism of nonthyroid origin with a defect in the maintenance of mitochondrial respiratory control. J. Clin. Invest. 41: 1776.

Lundberg, P., Stalberg, E., Thiele, B. 1974. Paralysis periodica paramyotonica. J. Neurol. Sci. 21: 309–321.

Magee, K. 1966. Paramyotonia congenita. Arch. Neurol. 14: 590–594.

Markand, O., D'Agostino, A. 1971. Ultrastructural changes in skeletal muscle induced by colchicine. Arch. Neurol. 24: 72–

Markand, O., North, R., D'Agostino, A., et al. 1969. Benign X-linked muscular dystrophy. Neurology 19: 617–633.

Markesbery, W., McQuillen, M., Proscopis, P., et al. 1974. Muscle carnitine deficiency. Arch. Neurol. 31: 320–324.

Mastaglia, F. 1973. Pathological changes in skeletal muscle in acromegaly. Acta Neuropathol. 24: 273–286.

Mastaglia, F., Barwick, D., Hall, R. 1970. Myopathy in acromegaly. Lancet 2: 907–909.

Mastaglia, F., Walton, J. 1970. Coxsacki virus-like particles in skeletal muscle from polymyositis. J. Neurol. Sci. 11: 593–599.

Mathew, N., Jacob, J., Chandy, J. 1970. Familial ocular myopathy and curare sensitivity. Arch. Neurol. 22: 68–74.

McArdle, B. 1951. Myopathy due to a defect in muscle glycogen breakdown. Clin. Sci. 10: 13–35.

McKeran, R., et al. 1980. Hypothyroid myopathy. A clinical and pathological study. J. Pathology 132: 35–54.

McQuillen, M., Johns, R. 1967. The nature of the defect in the Eaton-Lambert syndrome. Neurology 17: 527–536.

Mehler, M., Di Mauro, S. 1977. Residual acid maltase activity in late-onset maltase deficiency. Neurology 27: 178–184.

Melmed, C., Karpati, G., Carpenter, S. 1975. Experimental mitochondrial myopathy produced by in vivo uncoupling of oxidative phosphorylation. J. Neurol. Sci. 26: 305–318.

Meyers, K., et al. 1972. Periodic muscle weakness, normakolemia and tubular aggregates. Neurology 22: 269–279.

Mikol, J., Felten-Papaiconomou, A., Ferchal, F., et al. 1982. Inclusion body myositis: clinopathological studies and isolation of an adenovirus type 2 from muscle biopsy specimen. Ann. Neurol. 11: 576–581.

Miller, N., Moses, H. 1977. Ocular involvement in wound botulism. Arch. Ophthalmol. 95: 1788-1789.

Milstad, P., Bihmer, T. 1979. Transport of L-carnitine induced by prednisolone in an established cell line (CCL 27). A possible explanation of the therpeutic effect of glucocorticoids in muscular carnitine deficiency syndrome. Biochem. Biophys. Acta 585: 94–99.

Molenaar, P., Newsom-Davis, J., Polak, R., Vincent, A. 1982. Eaton-Lambert syndrome: Acetylcholine and choline acetyltransferase in skeletal muscle. Neurology 32: 1062–1065.

Mommaerts, W., Illingworth, B., Pearson, C., et al. 1959. A functional disorder of muscle associated with the absence of phosphorylase. Proc. Natl. Acad. Sci. 45: 791–797.

Morgan-Hughes, J., Darveniza, P., Landon, D. et al. 1979. A mitochondrial myopathy with deficiency of respiratory chain NADH-CoQ reductase activity. J. Neurol Sci. 43: 27.

Most, H. 1978. Trichinosis—Preventable, yet still with us. NEJM 298: 1178–1180.

Munsat, T. 1967. Therapy of myotonia. Neurology 17: 359–367.

Munsat, T., Piper, D., Cancilla, P., et al. 1972. Inflammatory myopathy with facioscapulohumeral distribution. Neurology 22: 335–347.

Murnaghan, M. 1960. Site and mechanism in tick paralysis. Science 131: 418–419.

Najjar, S. 1974. Muscular hypertrophy in hypothyroid children: The Kocher-Debré-Semelaigne syndrome. J. Pediatr. 85: 236–239.

Nelson, T., Flewellen, E. 1983. The malignant hyperthermia syndrome. NEJM 309: 416–418.

Niebroj-Dobosz, I. 1976. Erythrocyte ghosts (Na⁻K⁻) ATPase activity in Duchenne dystrophy and myotonia. J. Neurol. 214: 61–69.

Nori, M., Takamoti. 1976. Hyperthyroidism and myasthenia gravis with features of Eaton-Lambert syndrome. Neurology 26: 882–877.

Norris, F. 1966. Neuromuscular transmission in the thyroid disease. Ann. Intern. Med. 64: 81.

O'Grady, F., Smith, B. 1966. Neuromyopathy in the mouse produced by the antimicrobial agent mitroxoline. J. Path. Bact. 92: 43.

Olanow, W., Lane, R., Roses, A. 1982. Thymectomy in late-onset myasthenia gravis. Arch. Neurol. 39: 82-83.

Olson, B., Fenichel, G. 1982. Progressive muscle disease in a young woman with family history of Duchenne's muscular dystrophy. Arch. Neurol. 39: 378–380.

Olson, W., Engel, W. K., Walsh, G. et al. 1972. Oculocraniosomatic neuromuscular disease with "ragged-red" fibers. Arch. Neurol. 26: 193–211.

Osserman, K., Tsairis, P., Weiner, L. 1967. Myasthenia gravis and thyroid disease, clinical and immunologic correlation. J. Mount Sinai Hosp. N.Y. 34: 469–483.

Pande, S. 1975. A mitochondrial carnitine, acylcarnitine translocase system. Proc. Nat. Acad. Sci. 72: 883–877.

Patten, B. 1978. Myasthenia gravis: review of diagnosis and management. Muscle & Nerve 1: 190–205.

Patten, B., Bilezikian, J., Mallette, L., et al. 1974. Neuromuscular disease in primary hyperparathyroidism. Ann. Intern. Med. 80: 182–193.

Patterson, V., Hill, T., Fletcher, P., et al. 1979. Central core disease. Brain 102: 581–594.

Paulson, O., Engel, A. G., Gomez, M., 1974. Muscle blood flow in Duchenne type muscular dystrophy, limb-girdle dystrophy, polymyositis and in normal controls. JNNP 37: 685–690, 1974.

Pearson, C. 1964. The periodic paralysis: Differential features and pathological observations in permanent myopathic weakness. Brain 87: 341–354.

Pelligrini, G., Mosca, G., Cerri, C. 1978. Pompe's disease: ultrastructural alterations of muscle tissue in parents. Acta Neurol. Scand. 57: 216–222.

Percy, A., Miller, M. 1975. Reduced deformability of erythrocyte membranes from patients with Duchenne muscular dystrophy. Nature 258: 147–148.

Percy, M., Chan, L., Murphy, E. 1979. Serum creatine kinase and pyruvate kinase in Duchenne muscular dystrophy carrier detection. Muscle & Nerve 2: 329–339.

Perdoff, G. 1971. Alcoholic myopathy. Annu. Rev. Med. 22: 125–132.

Perkoff, G., Dioso, M., Bleisch, V., Klinkerfuss, G. 1967. A spectrum of myopathy associated with alcoholism (Part I) Ann. Intern. Med. 67: 481–492.

Perlo, V., et al. 1971. The role of thymectomy in the treatment of myasthenia gravis. Ann. N.Y. Acad. Sci. 183: 308–315.

Pickett, J., Layzer, R., Levin, S., Schneider, V., Campbell, M., Sumner, A. 1975. Neuromuscular complications of acromegaly. Neurology 25: 638–645.

Plishker, G., Gitelman, H., Appel, S. 1978. Myotonic muscular dystrophy: Altered calcium transport in erythrocytes. Science 200: 323–325.

Plorde, J. 1977. Harrison's Principles of Internal Medicine. New York: McGraw-Hill Book, pp. 1100–1102.

Polgar, J., et al. 1972. The early detection of dystrophia myotonica. Brain 95: 761–776.

Poser, E., Murphy, E., Thompson, M. 1969. Intelligence and the gene for muscular dystrophy. Arch. Dis. Child. 44: 221.

Poskanzer, D., Kerr, D. 1961. A third type of periodic paralysis with normokalemia and favorable response to sodium chloride. Am. J. Med. 31: 328–342.

Poskanzer, D., Kerr, D. 1961. Periodic paralysis with response to spironolactone. Lancet 2: 511–513.

Powell, L. 1953. Sarcoidosis of skeletal muscle. Am. J. Clin. Pathol. 23: 881–889.

Pryse-Phillips, W., Johnson, G., Chir, B., Larsen, B. 1982. Incomplete manifestations of myotonic dystrophy in a large kinship in Labrador. Ann. Neurol. 11: 582–591.

Ramsay, I. 1968. Thyrotoxic muscle disease. Postgrad. Med. J. 44: 383–397.

Rao, S., et al. 1980. Neuromuscular status in hypothyroidism. Acta Neurol. Scand. 61: 167–177.

Rebouche, C., Engel, A. 1983. Carnitine metabolism and deficiency syndromes. Mayo Clin. Proc. 58: 533–540.

Reza, M., Kar, N., Pearson, C., et al. 1978. Recurrent myoglobinuria due to muscle carnitine palmityl transferase deficiency. Ann. Intern. Med. 88: 610–615.

Riggs, J., Griggs, R., Moxley, R. 1977. Acetazolamide induced weakness in paramyotonia congenita. Ann. Intern. Med. 86: 169–173.

Ringel, S., Claman, H. 1982. Amyloid-associated muscle pseudohypertrophy. Arch. Neurol. 39: 413–417.

Rodnitzky, R., Goeken, J. 1982. Complications of plasma exchange in neurological patients. Arch. Neurol. 39: 350–354.

Rosenow, E., Engel, A. G. 1978. Acid maltase deficiency in adults presenting as respiratory failure. Am. J. Med. 64: 485–491.

Roses, A., Roses, M., Miller, S., et al. 1976. Carrier detection in Duchenne muscular dystrophy. NEJM 294: 193–198.

Roses, A., Roses, M., Nicholson, G., et al. 1977. Lactate dehydrogenase isoenzymes in detecting carriers of Duchenne muscular dystrophy. Neurology 27: 414–421.

Roses, M., Nicholson, M., Kirchner, C., et al. 1977. Evaluation and detection of Duchenne's and Becker's muscular dystrophy carriers by manual muscle testing. Neurology 27: 20–25.

Ross, R., 1963. Ocular myopathy sensitive to curare. Brain 86: 67–74.

Ross, B. et al. 1981. Examination of a case of suspected McArdle's syndrome by ^{31}P nuclear magnetic resonance. NEJM 304: 1338–1342.

Rothman, S., Bischoff, R. 1983. Electrophysiology of Duchenne dystrophy myotubes in tissue culture. Ann. Neurol. 13: 176–179.

Rowland, L. 1980. Biochemistry of muscle membranes in Duchenne muscular dystrophy. Muscle & Nerve 3: 3–20.

Rowland, L., 1980. Controversies about the treatment of myasthenia gravis. JNNP 43: 644–659.

Rowland, L., Fahn, S., Schotland, D. 1963. McArdle's disease. Arch. Neurol. 9: 325–342.

Rowland, L., Fetell, M., Olarte, M. et al. 1979. Emery-Dreifuss muscular dystrophy. Ann. Neurol. 5: 111–117.

Roy, S., Dubowitz, V. 1970. Carrier detection in Duchenne muscular dystrophy. J. Neurol Sci. 11: 65–79.

Rubenstein, A., Wainapel, S. 1977. Acute hypokalemic myopathy in alcoholism. Arch. Neurol. 34: 353–355.

Rubin, E. 1979. Alcoholic myopathy in heart and skeletal muscle. NEJM 301: 28–33.

Ruff, R., Secrist, D. 1982. Viral studies in benign acute childhood myositis. Arch. Neurol. 39: 261–263.

Salick, A., Pearson, C. 1967. Electrical silence of myoedema. Neurology. 17: 899–901.

Samaha, F. 1964. Von Eulenberg's paramyotonia. Trans. Am. Neurol. Assoc. 89: 87–91.

Satoyoshi, S., Kinoshita, M. 1977. Oculopharyngodistal myopathy. Arch. Neurol. 34: 89–92.

Satoyoshi, E., Murakami, K., Kowa, H. 1963. Myopathy of thyrotoxicosis. Neurology 13: 645–653.

Satyamurti, S., Drachman, D., Slone, F. 1975. Blockade of acetylcholine receptors, a model of myasthenia gravis. Science 187: 955–957.

Sawhney, B. et al. 1976. Pseudohypertrophic myopathy in cysticercosis. Neurology 26: 270–272.

Schiller, H., Stalberg, E. 1978. Human botulism studies with single fiber electromyography. Arch. Neurol. 35: 346–349.

Schmid, R., Mahler, R. 1959. Chronic progressive myopathy with myoglobinuria: demonstration of glycogenolytic defect in the muscle. J. Clin. Invest. 38: 2044–2058.

Schnitzler, E., Robertson, W. 1979. Familial Kearns-Sayre syndrome. Neurology 29: 1172–1174.

Schollmeyer, J., Goll, J., Robson, D., et al. 1973. Localization of alpha-actinin and tropomyosin in different muscles. J. Cell. Biol. 59: 306-A.

Schotland, D., Di Mauro, S., Bonilla, F. et al. 1976. Neuromuscular disorder associated with a defect in mitochondrial energy supply. Arch. Neurol. 33: 475.

Schraeder, P., Peters, H., Dahl, D. 1972. Polymyositis and penicillamine. Arch. Neurol. 27: 456-457.

Schwartz, G., Liu, C. 1954. Chronic progressive external ophthalmoplegia. A clinical and neuropathologic report. Arch. Neurol Psychiat. 71: 31–53.

Scott, W., Thalacker, J. 1981. Diagnosis and treatment of thyroid myopathy. Ophthalmology 88: 493–498.

Serratrice, G., Pellissier, J., 35 al. 1978. Centronuclear myopathy. Possible central nervous system origin. Muscle & Nerve 1: 62–69.

Seybould, M., Drachman, D. 1974. Gradually increasing doses of prednisone in myasthenia gravis. NEJM 290: 81-84.

Sghirlanzoni, A., Peluchetti, D., Mantegazza, R., et al, 1984. Myasthenia gravis: Prolonged treatment with steroids, Neurology 34: 170-174.

Sher, J., Rimalovski, A., Athanassiadas, T., et al. 1967. Familial centronuclear myopathy. Neurology 17: 727–742.

Shumate, J., Katnik, R., Ruiz, M. et al. 1979. Myoadenylate deaminase deficiency. Muscle & Nerve 2: 213–216.

Shy, G., Engel, W. K., Somers, J., et al. 1963. Nemaline myopathy. Brain 86: 793–810.

Shy, G., Magee, K. 1956. A new congenital non-progressive myopathy. Brain 79: 610–621.

Siegel, I. 1978. The management of muscular dystrophy: A clinical review. Muscle & Nerve 1: 453–460.

Simon, D., Ringel, S., Sufit, R., 1982. Clinical spectrum of fascial inflammation. Muscle & Nerve 5: 525–537.

Simpson, J. 1978. Myasthenia gravis: a personal view of pathogenesis and mechanism. Muscle & Nerve 1: 45–56, 151–156.

Skinner, R., Smith, C., Emery, A. 1974. Linkage between the loci for benign (Becker-type) X-borne muscular dystrophy and deutan colour blindness. J. Med. Genet. 11: 317–320.

Slonim, A., Borum, P., Mrak, R. et al. 1983. Nonketotic hypoglycemia: an early indicator of systemic carnitine deficiency. Neurology 33: 29–34.

Slonim, A., Coleman, R., McElligot, M. et al. 1983. Improvement of muscle function in acid maltase deficiency by high protein diet therapy.Neurology 33: 3436.

Smith, A., MacFie, W., Oliver, M. 1970. Clofibrate, serum enzymes and muscle pain. Brit. Med. J. 2: 86.

Smith, B., O'Grady, F. 1966. Experimental chloroquine myopathy. JNNP 29: 235-258.

Smith, R., Stern, G. 1967. Myopathy, osteomalacia, and hyperparathyroidism. Brain 90: 593-602.

Solemon, D., Bennett, L., Brown, J., et al. 1968. Hyperthyroidism. Ann. Intern. Med. 69: 1015-1017.

Spiro, A., Moore, C., Prineas, J. et al. 1970. A cytochrome related inherited disorder of the nervous system and muscle. Arch. Neurol. 23: 103.

Spiro, A., Shy, M., Gonatas, N. 1966. Myotubular myopathy. Arch. Neurol. 14: 1-14.

Sulaiman, W., Doyle, W., Johnson, R., et al. 1974. Myopathy with mitochondrial inclusion bodies: Histological and metabolic studies. JNNP 37: 1236-1246.

Takamori, M., Ishii, N., Muri, M. 1973. The role of cyclic $3'$, $5'$−adrenosine monophosphate in neuromuscular transmission. Arch. Neurol. 29: 420–424.

Takeuchi, A., Takeuchi, N. 1960. On the permeability of the end plate membrane during the action of transmitter. J. Physiol. 154: 52–67.

Tarui, S., Kono, N., Nasu, T., 35 al. 1969. Enzymatic basis for the coexistence of myopathy and hemolytic disease in inherited muscle phosphofructokinase deficiency. Biochem. Biophys. Res. Commun. 34: 77–83.

Tarui, S., Okono, G., Ikura, Y., et al. 1965. Phosphofructokinase deficiency in skeletal muscle: A new kind of glycogenosis. Biochem. Biophys. Res. Commun. 19: 517–523.

Telerman-Toppet, N., Gerard, J., Coers, C. 1973. Central core disease: A study of clinically unaffected muscle. J. Neurol. Sci. 19: 207–223.

Teravainen, H., Larsen, A. 1977. Some features of the neuromuscular complications of pulmonary carcinoma. Ann. Neurol. 2: 495–502.

Thompson, B., Corbett, J., Thompson, S. 1982. Pseudo-Horner's syndrome, Arch Neurol. 39: 108-111.

Tornheim, K., Lowenstein, J. 1974. The purine nucleotide cycle: interactions with oscillations of the glycolytic pathway in muscle extracts. J. Biol. Chem. 249: 3241-3246.

Van Haeverbeek, M., Ectors, M., VanHaelst, L., Franken, L. 1974. Myopathy caused by polymyxin E. JNNP 37: 1343.

Van Winjngaarden, G., Bethlem, J. 1971. The facioscapulohumeral syndrome. In Kakulas, B. (ed). *Proceedings of the Second International Congress on Muscle Disease* (abstr.). Amsterdam: Excepta Medica, p. 54.

Venables, G., Bates, D., Shaw, D. 1978. Hypothyroidism with true myotonia. JNNP 41: 1013-1015.

Vignos, P., Greene, R. 1973. Oxidative respiration of skeletal muscle in experimental corticosteroid myopathy. J. Lab. Clin. Med. 81: 365-378.

Vignus, P., Spencer, G., Archibald, K. 1963. Management of progressive muscular dystrophy of childhood. JAMA 184: 89-96.

Viskoper, R., et al. 1973. Acetazolamide treatment in hypokalemic periodic paralysis. Am. J. Med. Sci. 266: 119-123.

Vroom, F., Jarrell, M., Maren, T. 1975. Acetazolamide treatment of hypokalemic paralysis. Neurology 32: 385–392.

Walton, J. 19 . Disorders of Voluntary Muscle. New York: Churchill Livingstone, pp. 684–688.

Wang, P., Clausen, T. 1976. Treatment of attacks in familial hyperkalemic periodic paralysis by inhalation of salbutamol. Lancet 1: 221–223.

Weber, L., Nashel, D., Mellow, M. 1981. Pharyngeal dysphagia in alcoholic myopathy. Ann. Intern. Med. 95: 189–191.

Whelan, J. 1980. Baclofen in the treatment of the stiff-man syndrome. Arch. Neurol. 37: 600–601.

Whisnant, J. 1963. Chloroquine neuromyopathy. Mayo Clin. Proc. 38: 501–513.

Whitaker, J. 1982. Inflammatory myopathy. A review of etiologic and pathogenic factors. Muscle & Nerve 5: 573–592.

Williams, R. 1959. Triamcinolone myopathy. Lancet 1: 698–701.

Willner, J., Ginsburg, S., Di Mauro, S. 1978. Active transport of carnitine into skeletal muscle. Neurology 721-724.

Willner, J., Wood, D., Cerri, C., et al. 1980. Increased myophosphorylase A in malignant hyperthermia. NEJM 303: 138-140.

Winer, N., et al. 1965. Induced myotonia in man and goats. J. Lab. Clin. Med. 66: 758.

Winters, S., et al. 1976. Familial mitral valve prolapse and myotonic dystrophy. Ann. Intern. Med. 85: 19-22.

Woolf, A. 1966. Morphology of the myasthenic neuromuscular junction. Ann. N.Y. Acad. Sci. 135: 35-58.

Zellweger, H., Jonasescu, V. 1973. Myotonic dystrophy and its differential diagnosis. Acta Neurol. Scand. (Supp. 55) 49: 5-28.

Index

Acetylcholine, 25, 41, 43, 44, 47, 52
Acetylcholine receptor protein, 41, 58
Acetylcholine receptor antibody, 58,
    62, 63–64
Acetylcholinesterase, 43
Acid maltase, 166
Acid maltase deficiency, 2, 5, 25, 145,
    166–169
  adult, 166–169
  clinical presentation, 166–167
  electromyography, 168
  infantile, 166
  muscle biopsy, 167–168
  pathophysiology, 169
  serum muscle enzymes, 167
  treatment, 169
Acromegaly, 191–193
Acute idiopathic polyneuropathy,
    see Guillain-Barré syndrome
Acute intermittent porphyria and
    polyneuropathy, 3, 6 124
Adynamia episodica hereditaria, see
    Hyperkalemic periodic paralysis
Alcoholic myopathy, 2, 5, 6, 7, 9, 13,
    14, 205–209
  clinical presentation, 205–207
  laboratory studies, 208–209
  pathogenesis, 209
Amyotrophic lateral sclerosis, 194
Anterior horn cell disease, 3, 5, 7, 14
Antibiotics contraindicated in myas-
    thenia gravis, 65

Becker's muscular dystrophy, see
    Benign x-linked muscular
    dystrophy (Becker type)
Benign x-linked muscular dystrophy
    (Becker type), 5, 79–81
  carrier detection, 81–82
  clinical presentation, 79–81
  electrodiagnostic testing, 81
  muscle biopsy, 81
  serum muscle enzymes, 81
  treatment, 81
Benign x-linked muscular dystrophy
    (Emery-Dreifuss type), 82–83
Beta-Oxidation of fatty acids, 178
Biopsy, see specific disorder
Botulism, 4, 6, 13, 14, 50–53, 124
  clinical presentation, 50–51
  electrodiagnostic tests, 51
  muscle biopsy, 51
  serum muscle enzymes, 51
  pathophysiology, 52
  treatment and prognosis, 52–53

Carcinoma and myositis, 143, 144
Carnitine, 177, 178
Carnitine deficiency, 2, 5, 6, 145
    178, 179–184
  blood studies, 180
  case report, 183–184
  clinical presentation, 179–180
  electrodiagnostic studies, 180
  muscle biopsy, 150, 181

235

[Myotonic atrophy]
  neonatal, 109, 114–116
  serum muscle enzymes, 112
  summary, 115
  treatment, 113–114
Myotonic dystrophy, *see* Myotonic
  atrophy
Myotubular myopathy, *see* Type I
  fiber hypotrophy with central
  nuclei

NADH coenzyme Q reductase deficiency, 187
Nemaline myopathy, *see* Rod
  disease
Neuropathies, 2, 3, 5, 7, 8, 12, 13, 25,
  145, 191
Neuromuscular junction, 17
  anatomy and physiology, 41–44
  diseases, 44–72
Normokalemic periodic paralysis, 131,
  132, 133

Ocular muscle weakness, 4, 13–14
Oculopharyngeal dystrophy, 2, 4, 5,
  13
  clinical presentation, 83–84
  laboratory studies, 84–85
  pathophysiology, 85
  treatment, 85

Pain, *see* Muscle discomfort
Palpation
  of muscle, 13
  of nerves, 13
Paramyotonic congenita, 16, 118–121
  clinical presentation, 118–120
  laboratory studies, 120–121
  treatment, 121
Paraneoplastic neuropathies, 3, 6
Percussion of muscles, 16
Periodic paralysis, 5, 6, 14, 16, 123–
  132
  see also Hyperkalemic periodic
  paralysis, Hypokalemic periodic
  paralysis, and Normokalemic
  periodic paralysis
Phosphofructokinase, 161
Phosphofructokinase deficiency, 166
  clinical presentation, 175–176

[Phosphofructokinase deficiency]
  laboratory studies, 176
  pathophysiology, 176
  treatment, 177
Physical examination, 12–16
Plexopathies, 3
Polymyalgia rheumatica, 8, 9, 13, 153
Polymyositis, 2, 4, 5, 6, 8, 9, 14, 107,
  144–149, 167
  case report, 149
  clinical presentation, 144
  electromyography, 145, 147
  muscle biopsy, 145–146
  neoplasms with, 143
  pathogenesis, 147
  serum muscle enzymes, 145
  summary, 150
  treatment, 147–149
Pompe's disease, *see* Acid maltase
  deficiency, infantile
Popeye arm, 88
Pseudocontracture, 7
Ptosis, 4, 13–14

Ragged red fiber disease, 2, 5, 13,
  188–190
  clinical presentation, 188–189
  laboratory, 188, 189–190
  pathophysiology, 190
  treatment, 190
Reflexes, 16
Regional curare test, 64–65
Rod disease, 3, 5, 91, 101–104
  clinical presentation, 101–102
  electrodiagnostic tests, 103
  muscle biopsy, 102–103
  pathophysiology, 104
  serum muscle enzymes, 103
  treatment, 104

Sarcoid myopathy, 2, 145, 153–
  157
  clinical presentation, 153–155
  laboratory studies, 155
  pathogenesis, 155
  summary, 156
  treatment, 157
Schwartz–Jampel syndrome, 107
Second wind phenomenon, 164,
  170